THE NEW BODY TALK

The New
Body Talk

Self-help for all
your health problems

Michael van Straten

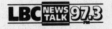

HEADLINE

First published as *Body Talk* in 1987
by J. M. Dent & Sons Ltd

This edition first published in 1993
by HEADLINE BOOK PUBLISHING PLC

10 9 8 7 6 5 4 3 2 1

ISBN 0 7472 4156 2

Typeset by Keyboard Services, Luton

Printed and bound in Great Britain by
HarperCollins Manufacturing, Glasgow

HEADLINE BOOK PUBLISHING PLC
Headline House
79 Great Titchfield Street
London W1P 7FN

Contents

List of illustrations

This book is dedicated to three teachers: the late Monty Fry, who taught me how to learn; the late Dr Norman Knox, who taught me about 'proper doctoring'; and the late Bagnall-Goodwin, whose kindness helped me and many others through our college years

For my children, Sacha and Tanya

Acknowledgements

The author and publishers would like to thank Macdonald & Company (Publishers) Ltd for permission to quote from *The Allergy Diet* by Elizabeth Workman, Dr John Hunter and Dr Virginia Alun Jones.

Foreword

It's now six years since I wrote the first edition of *Body Talk*, and in that time more has changed in the world of complementary medicine than in the previous sixty. During the mid 1980s there was a growing trend towards a wider acceptance of therapies like osteopathy, chiropractic, acupuncture, homoeopathy and herbal medicine. Now as we move towards the middle 90s it's not just the public who are seeking out gentler, less invasive and more patient-friendly treatments but health-care professionals across the board of orthodox medicine who are also getting more involved.

There is a thirst for knowledge among public and practitioners alike, and both professional and lay magazines are full of small ads for seminars, workshops, symposia and training courses. From reflexology to aromatherapy, from massage to meditation, from healing to herb gardens, the choice is seemingly endless. Last year I was asked by the Lisa Sainsbury Foundation to give a series of one-day seminars in hospitals in London and the south of England. The Foundation provides educational seminars for hospital staff caring for terminally ill patients and it had received a number of requests for more information on complementary medicine. Working with these remarkable nurses was one of the most rewarding things I have ever done. We started each day with a discussion about the information that they would find most useful, and without exception all the groups chose nutrition, massage and relaxation techniques as the subjects which would enable them to give better care to their patients.

In the world of high-tech medicine these carers knew that the touch of another human, above all, could bring ease and comfort to the desperately sick in intensive care units, acute surgical wards, to the very young, to the very old and to cancer and AIDS patients.

The academic standards of training have risen dramatically, especially in osteopathy where the principal schools have come to-gether to form a joint registration body to ensure the highest possible quality of graduates. The British School of Osteopathy, the British College of Naturopathy and Osteopathy, and the European College of Chiropractic have all achieved BSc degree status for their courses, and in spite of the present financial situation the number of applicants for these courses is growing. Many would-be students come straight from school with A levels, and many turn later to complementary medicine as a career, as a result of their own experiences.

Many parents, who in the past may have been dubious about their children taking this unorthodox path, are now more accepting since their offspring will complete their training with a recognised science degree. The next vital step is a State Register, and this is just around the corner. The committee set up by the King's Fund to study osteopathy concluded that there should be a statutory register of osteopaths. A bill is already before Parliament and looks likely to become law. Certainly other therapies will take this route as they become more harmonised and are able to establish the requisite academic standards of professional ability and safety.

Why, you may ask, do complementary practitioners want to be registered and regulated? The truth is that many don't. It is in the public's interest that this should happen, firstly because it will provide a measure of protection against the confidence tricksters, quacks and charlatans who are jumping on the bandwagon of complementary medicine, and secondly because it will make these therapies more widely available within the framework of the NHS. It has always seemed iniquitous to me that we all pay for the Health Service – it has never been 'free' – and yet the choice of treatment has excluded complementary medicine. There are already acupuncturists working in hospital pain clinics, osteopaths and chiropractics holding clinics in some NHS GP surgeries, masseurs and aromatherapists working in cancer units. Statutory recognition can only increase the possibilities of more complementary medicine freely available to more people.

Even private health insurance companies now recognise some therapies as specialist treatment and are prepared to pay for them. More and more employers provide osteopathy, massage and relaxation therapy for their workforce, and as the mounting toll of RSI – repetitive strain injury – becomes a major factor in absenteeism, compensation cases and, worst of all, pain and suffering, companies are turning to osteopaths and chiropractors for advice on seating, workstations and office practices.

After more than ten years of broadcasting and writing I am still surprised by the public response to health information. Sackfuls of letters still pour in to LBC requesting diet sheets, leaflets, fact sheets and other information, and a recent offer of a healthy cookery booklet in my weekly Body Talk column for the *Sunday People* brought in 15,000 requests. There is no doubt in my mind that the impact of complementary medicine will continue to grow. More and more people will try self-help and more and more people will seek professional help. But the most exciting thing of all is the prospect of patients being offered complementary therapy as a matter of course when they consult their own GPs.

It won't happen tomorrow, it won't happen next month and it probably won't happen next year, but I am sure it will happen before the end of the decade.

How to use this book

This is not a medical textbook. You will not find endless lists of strange and rare diseases nor will you find an authoritative text on complementary therapies. After five years of phone-in programmes and two years of Body Talk on LBC I have become aware of a very definite pattern which clearly defines the areas of health problems which most concern you, the public. Week in and week out the same type of problems crop up on the phone-in programmes and in the thousand or so letters which I receive every single week. Some of these problems relate to serious and even occasionally life-threatening diseases, but the vast majority of them are concerned with very common problems which are not always well treated by the orthodox medical profession.

From back ache to bunions, from constipation to catarrh, from cramp to cystitis, these are the everyday complaints for which this book will provide some of the answers. 'You have to learn to live with it', 'What do you expect at your age?', 'Well, it won't kill you'. These are the sort of expressions which make me see red and the sort of expressions which patients all too commonly hear from their medical practitioners. The age question is particularly true with women. So many problems which women suffer from are attributed to menstruation, menopause, premenstrual tension, post-menstrual problems, when more often than not there are very specific physical reasons for them. As for the seriousness of any medical problem, for me the sole criterion of seriousness is whether or not it prevents the patient from leading a full, normal and active life.

To the concert pianist a rose thorn in the finger is a disaster; to the professional footballer an ingrowing toenail could mean weeks away from his game; to the busy mother back ache can be an overwhelming problem which stops her lifting the baby out of the cot or going to do the shopping; and for the pensioner a corn on the foot can make walking so difficult as to immobilise an otherwise healthy and active person. Any problem, no matter how minor in the scale of life to death, which interferes with your activity and your lifestyle and your ability to pursue successfully your chosen occupation, is a disaster.

The object of this book is to help people help themselves to better health. It seldom provides all the answers but nearly always will give you guidelines as to measures that you can take to help your body recover more quickly from any ailment.

Holistic medicine is a term which embraces the overall concept of complementary therapies. The truly holistic practitioner must regard his patient as a trilogy of body, mind and spirit and furthermore must also take into account the environment within which that person works and lives. Whilst the true concept of holism is one in which you treat the patient and not the disease, one in which we despise the 'pill for every ill' approach to medical care, there are many specific measures that can be taken to alleviate the immediate discomfort of problems whilst giving you time to pursue the overall object of a holistic approach to eradicating the cause as well as treating the uncomfortable symptoms. The conditions and symptoms discussed in the book are arranged according to the system of the body which they affect so that asthma, bronchitis, and coughs appear in the respiratory system, whilst arthritis, back pain, fibrositis and tennis elbow appear in the muscle, joint and skeletal system. Likewise, anorexia, depression and insomnia appear under the nervous system, with psoriasis, shingles, eczema occurring in the skin section, and so on throughout the book. In addition to a brief description of each condition, you will find listed things which you can do for yourself to relieve the problem and also, where applicable, the sort of complementary practitioner that would be most likely to offer you satisfactory treatment for your particular problem.

In sickness and in health

Looking back, it is easy to see how people get hooked on pethidine, the injection you get before an operation. As you lie in the twilight world between reality and unconsciousness, everything seems far away: sounds, smells, sights – everything, that is, except the gnawing fear. The fear of yet another operation, the fear of the mask closing over your face, the awful smell of rubber, the fear of waking up in pain, the fear of the endless vomiting, the fear of the daily visit by the surgeon to change dressings congealed with blood that sticks to each molecule of skin. The fear of not waking up at all. Yet all is dulled and pushed into the very deepest recesses of the conscious mind by the miracle of pethidine.

Forty years later, I can still close my eyes and relive each agonising experience, for in those days I was a sickly and ailing child, in and out of hospital, with countless trips to Harley Street, the Mecca of medical excellence and the haunt of unscrupulous charlatans, and repeated encounters with the surgeons and anaesthetists. I can remember the starchy rustle of the nurses' uniforms, the endless routine of life in a large teaching hospital, the ward rounds, the whispered decisions taken at the foot of the bed, the bustling and always cheerful matron, the quiet stillness of the dim night light casting a halo around the night nurse as she sat at the desk where she could see every bed.

To a seven-year-old, the world of medicine seemed magical. At this point I resolved to be a doctor. I wanted to repay the dedication, skill and kindness that had undoubtedly saved my life. To repay the debt which was owed to the remarkable men and women and of course to my parents who had sacrificed so much. There was no National Health Service in those days.

By 1957, I was set on the path to medical school, but then spent a year working as an orderly at a famous hospital where I soon became disillusioned with my romantic images of modern medicine. The system was beginning to take over. Yes, there were dedicated and brilliant doctors, caring nurses and remarkable results. But the patients were starting to be treated like symptoms not people. The drug industry was promoting the 'pill for every ill' concept of treatment and there seemed less and less time for that most important prescription of all, the one elixir that I had been given in enormous quantities as a child, Tender Loving Care.

These doubts were growing into a serious problem. A chance meeting with an old friend turned my steps towards alternative medicine. Donald had given up his highly promising career in science to become an osteopath. On an instant impulse, I gave up all thoughts of studying medicine and went to join my friend. This chance meeting altered the whole course of my life. It led me into new and unorthodox fields, and without recourse to the scalpel, dangerous drugs or invasive therapies, has allowed me to spend more than twenty years helping other people towards a healthier and more fulfilled life.

I have always been thankful for that chance meeting and for my impulsive decision. My therapeutic horizons have since broadened to include naturopathy, acupuncture and many other aspects of alternative medicine. This book is a distillation of things I have learned from teachers, practitioners, experience and, above all, from the many thousands of patients who have seen fit to visit me.

The consumer-led revolution

In 1959, when I first decided to become an osteopath, all those about me, including my student friends and my parents, thought that I had taken leave of my senses. After all, osteopathy was part of fringe medicine and certainly well beyond the pale of any orthodox beliefs. Today, some quarter of a century later, alternative medicine, or, as I prefer to call it, complementary medicine, has assumed the mantle of respectability. Even Prince Charles and other members of the Royal Family are known to favour homoeopathy and, in a speech as President of the British Medical Association, Prince Charles urged members of the orthodox medical profession to take more note of alternatives, especially healing, herbal medicine, acupuncture and osteopathy.

The media is full of tips on health care based on alternative medicine. The British Medical Association and the General Medical Council acknowledge the value of therapies such as osteopathy and acupuncture, and members of the general public have voted with their feet and moved their allegiance in their thousands from conventional, orthodox medicine towards the overall philosophy of a more natural approach to the treatment of disease.

What has caused this fundamental change in public opinion? There is no doubt that the public are better informed than they ever were before about medical matters. People are no longer content to go to the doctor and say, 'Please, doctor, do something'. They are much more likely to say, 'Please will you tell me what I can do to help myself with this particular problem'.

The thalidomide affair resulted in thousands of deformed babies being born. The continual stories of the side effects of drugs, mismanaged surgery, wrong limbs and organs being removed have all made the public far more conscious of their own responsibility in relation to health care. For this very reason, more and more people are seeking help from practitioners of complementary medicine. The patient is no longer satisfied merely to have his symptom treated. He wants to be treated in a much more holistic fashion. What is meant by holistic medicine? It has become a much abused and much quoted term but is very seldom applied in its correct form. To be holistic the practitioner has to consider the patient as a trilogy. He or she has to consider the body, mind and spirit and all these three in relationship to environment, work, family, psychological make-up and every single other factor which can impinge on that patient's life in any way whatsoever.

As conventional medicine becomes more and more technological, the specialist becomes a practitioner who tends to be interested more and more in less and less. One can easily foresee the situation where one consults a specialist for the left ear and another for the right, and neither of them looks at the head that separates the ears, or the body that carries the head.

A fundamental concept of nearly all of the complementary therapies is that of holism. You cannot take symptoms in isolation from the patient and treat them one at a time. Unless the practitioner is prepared to look at the entire patient as a whole living, functioning organism, all he is doing is alleviating the symptoms and doing nothing to treat 'the patient'.

Moving a step further, it is plain that even treating the patient as a whole is not enough if you are to do more than remove the symptoms of his complaint. In order to achieve long-term results, it is vital that the practitioner should play an important part in helping to re-educate the patient to change his lifestyle, and to prevent the conditions arising which lead to the symptoms from which the patient is complaining. For example, no naturopath faced with a patient suffering from high blood pressure would be doing his job properly if he did not investigate fully the patient's lifestyle. Does he drink; does he smoke; does he know how to relax; does he take exercise; what does he eat; what sort of job does he do? How are the relations within his family, his personal life? All these factors play an important role in the origins of high blood pressure and no matter what herbs you prescribe, no matter what specific diets are suggested, unless you can help that patient to readjust his way of living, he will always have a problem with his high blood pressure. In the same way, the osteopath who sees a patient with back problems and does not teach the patient how to use his body, how to lift, how to sit, how to work, does not inquire what sort of work the patient does, does not encourage the patient to maintain healthy weight – that practitioner is falling down on the job.

Today, there are many orthodox doctors who have a growing interest in the various therapies of complementary medicine. But sadly, they seem to use these therapies in just the same way as they use their prescription pads. The pill for every ill becomes the diet for every disease, the manipulation for every malfunction, or the pin for every pain. These doctors frequently do short weekend courses in complementary therapies and have no conception whatsoever of the underlying philosophy, the thread of which runs like an endless stream of life throughout alternative medicine.

What is truly remarkable is that whilst the medical professionals have for many years decried the practices of the alternative therapists, little by little many of the concepts of naturopathy, acupuncture and herbal medicine have gradually drifted across the borders and have become common usage amongst doctors. Twenty-five years ago, as a student, I was faced with my first patient suffering from the distressing complaint of diverticulitis. In those days, the standard medical treatment was for the patient to avoid at all cost fibrous foods, wholemeal bread, roughage, vegetables, fruits, salads and to live entirely on a diet of bland food, milk puddings, steamed fish, boiled white rice. Coming face to face with a six-foot burly East End lorry driver suffering from diverticulitis was surely a test of the teachings which I had been exposed to at the British College of Naturopathy and Osteopathy. My first real patient for whom I was responsible and here was I about to give him advice which was totally contrary to that which he had been given by a famous surgeon at one of the country's leading teaching hospitals. 'Throw away your bag of sweets in the cab,' I said. 'Keep away from boiled fish, white rice, white bread, and change your diet immediately. You should eat only wholemeal bread, brown rice, lots of vegetables, lots of raw salads.' These were the very foods which his doctor had warned him could not only aggravate his disease but could lead to fatal consequences.

A few months later, I received a letter from this particular patient's consultant. He had been for his regular check-up at the hospital and told the doctor just what he could do with his boiled fish. After he had changed to my diet, his condition had completely resolved. The consultant wrote to me in the most aggressive terms: 'This patient,' he said, 'will surely die and I will see to it that you are in the coroner's court when it happens.' Happily the patient lived healthily and on a good balanced diet for many years to follow and to the best of my knowledge is still doing the same thing. Today every medical textbook suggests high fibre diets, plenty of roughage, plenty of vegetables, plenty of fruit, plenty of salads and above all the magical bran. Of course, many doctors prefer their patients to take the bran in tablet form, since this has a more scientific ring to it, rather than just telling them to eat wholemeal bread.

Another clear example of the way in which our therapies have crossed the borderline is that of food allergies. I was taught as a student that many illnesses, for example migraine, could be caused by the patient's reaction to some foods which did not agree with that individual's metabolism. In the case of migraine the most common foods that trigger an attack are cheese, chocolates, oranges, coffee, cocoa, and alcohol, especially red wines. The doctors pooh-poohed this idea and many of my patients were scorned by their general practitioners when they told them what I had suggested. However, for many people suffering from this distressing illness, it works. Today, there are migraine clinics in most big hospitals, all of which recommend dietary changes in order to promote relief from migraine attacks.

One only has to compare the foods available in health food stores today with those that are being sold in every supermarket throughout the country. Twenty years ago yoghurt, muesli, wholemeal bread, foods without preservatives, colourings and artificial additives, pulses and vegetarian dishes were all the exclusive preserve of the health food store. Today, not only can you find these foods in every supermarket throughout the land, but supermarkets are now even advertising themselves as the health food store near to you. They are changing their attitude because you, the customer, have forced them to do it. You see whole sections of healthier foods available in the supermarkets, which vie with one another to give better nutritional labelling information to the customers. The supermarket shelves are lined with products starkly labelled 'free from additives', 'free from colourings', 'free from preservatives'. The racks bulge with lentils, beans, dried fruits, herb teas, decaffeinated coffee, coffee substitutes and so on.

All this was unthinkable twenty years ago. So much so, that at that time when I was president of the Health Food Manufacturers' Association I dared, in a speech, to suggest that I looked forward to a time when there was no longer a need for health food stores as such and every supermarket would be a health food store. This statement was not popular in the health food industry, but happily the prophecy has come true and it is now possible for every man, woman and child in this country to buy healthier food in the supermarket.

Of course, there is a long way to go before we can winkle out all the facts from the big food manufacturers. They are reluctant to provide fuller labelling information on their packages. And for good reason. Their arguments are always that the housewife wouldn't understand the long words and would only be more confused if packages were labelled more fully. This is a gross underestimation of the intelligence of the average British shopper.

In my practice and in the Body Talk radio programme and the phone-in programmes that I do for LBC we are constantly reminded of how aware the public has become of the foods which they buy every day. They want to know how much fat there is in a sausage. They want to know how much real meat there is in a meat pie. I am sure that many of you are unaware of the fact that a meat pie can be labelled with meat content without differentiating between meat, fat, skin, gristle or bone that might or might not be in the pie. More and more mothers are becoming aware of the highly toxic effects of many of the food additives which are used in the food processing industry.

The industry claims that it is impossible to prove that many of these things are actually harmful. I maintain that manufacturers should be forced to prove that their products are safe before we expose ourselves and, more importantly, our children or even a baby in the mother's womb to the toxic hazards of these chemicals. One only has to look at the huge success of Maurice Hanssen's book *E for Additives*, which was in the best seller lists for weeks in the United Kingdom, to see how aware the British buying public has become of the dangers of what goes into the food that they eat every day.

In their book *The Food Scandal*, Caroline Walker and Geoffrey Cannon quote a remarkable statement made by Senator McGovern in the United States in 1977. He said, 'The simple fact is that our diets have changed radically within the last fifty years with great and very often harmful effects on our health. Too much fat, too much sugar or salt can be, and are, linked directly to heart disease, cancer, obesity and stroke, among other killer diseases. Those of us within government have an obligation to acknowledge this. The public wants some guidance, wants to know the truth.' As a young student I once heard Stanley Lief, the founder of Champneys, probably the most famous British health resort, and a formidable pioneer of naturopathy and osteopathy in this country, say he believed that the British people were digging their graves with their teeth. It took the government until 1979 to set up the National Advisory Committee on Nutrition Education. The resulting report from this committee, now known as the NACNE Report, was in fact finished early in 1981 but the government had been persuaded not to publish their findings. After all, there were huge vested interests at stake: those of the food combines involved in the production of fats and sugars, the dairy farmers, the meat producers and the giant sugar corporations. It was not until 3 July 1983 that *The Sunday Times* leaked the story to the general public.

For those of us in the naturopathic profession, the NACNE

Report seemed *déjà vu*. These things which we had all been preaching for years upon years upon years were suddenly pronounced by government scientists to be the truth. We were the ones who had been ridiculed for daring to suggest that people should eat less meat, daring to suggest that people should consume less dairy products, daring to suggest that wholemeal bread untampered with and unadulterated was healthier than white bread, the white bread so dearly beloved of the government because they controlled the added constituents that went into it.

In the autumn of 1992 the Health Education Authority launched a campaign called Enjoy Healthy Eating, backed up with a booklet of the same title. The HEA joined forces with supermarkets and leading food manufacturers to promote the campaign which, sadly, received very little media attention and seemed to pass largely unnoticed. Unfortunately the money available from the government to promote healthy eating is probably less for a whole year than the food industry spends in one week advertising high fat, high sugar, junk foods to our children.

To coincide with the campaign I was asked by Quaker Oats to do a round-Britain tour of radio stations promoting the idea of using oats – truly one of nature's superfoods – as part of a healthy eating regime. You can imagine how pleased I was to see the government spending its money – or rather, our money – encouraging people to adopt virtually all the good nutritional ideas which I and my colleagues have been advising as naturopaths for decades. The booklet stresses the importance of vitamins, minerals, good carbohydrates, fresh fruit, vegetables and salads, and warns about the dangers of excessive amounts of fats, salt and sugar in the diet.

This list looks like an extract from a naturopathic textbook of the 1930s. It says, eat more fibre, buy wholemeal bread, use wholemeal flour for pastry and pancakes. Use brown rice and wholemeal pasta. Eat more main dishes based on high fibre foods, rice, potatoes, beans, pasta and vegetables. Use rolled oats for crunchy topping. Cut down on fat. Choose lean cuts of meat and eat smaller portions. Trim off all the fat you can see. Grill rather than fry and drain off excess fat. Eat fish and poultry rather than red meat or made-up meat products. Buy skimmed or semi-skimmed milk. Use plain yoghurt instead of cream. Buy low fat cheeses – cottage cheese, Edam and Camembert – instead of high fat ones – like cream cheese or Cheddar or Stilton. Spread the butter or margarine thinly. Cut bread and chips thicker, so there is less surface area for fats. Cut down on fats in recipes. Use lentils to stretch or substitute for meat. Cut down on sugar. Have fresh fruit sometimes for pudding. Buy fruit tinned in natural juices. Halve the sugar in all recipes – it works for everything except ices. Cut down on confectionery, cakes, sweets, drinks and snacks. Cut down on salt. Reduce cooking salt.

Don't put salt on the table. Cut down on snacks and convenience foods with a high salt content. Cut down on highly salted crisps, nuts and other nibbles.

It is undoubtedly true to say that following this advice, advice that has been given over the years by the naturopaths, would change the health of our nation. If every mother today only fed her family on wholemeal bread, in two decades bowel disease would decline, especially if this change was accompanied by a reduction in the amount of red meat and a reduction in the huge quantities of dairy produce consumed in this country. Reducing the consumption of alcohol and encouraging young people to eat a more balanced, healthier diet, especially at schools and colleges, would make a huge difference. I have always thought it a great shame that children are not taught more about human nutrition and human anatomy and physiology at school rather than concentrating on the humble earthworm or dogfish. How much more sense it would make to teach youngsters to cook with wholemeal ingredients, to understand balanced diets and to use the infinitely cheaper but just as nutritious vegetable protein sources rather than the more expensive and potentially health-damaging meat products. Of course, it is not essential to be a vegetarian to remain healthy, but there is no doubt that a trend towards more vegetable protein and less animal protein in our national diet would have highly beneficial long-term effects. And wouldn't it make more sense to teach young people these facts rather than the rather pointless exercise of making iced fairy cakes, scones or sticky buns, to say nothing of starchy, fatty puddings and pies?

Since we are what we eat, and more and more of you are coming to realise that fact, it is hardly surprising that the medical profession feels itself somewhat in a state of siege. It is interesting that nutrition does not appear on the medical schools' syllabus at most universities, and if it does, it deals only with the gross deficiency diseases, which most practitioners in this country are unlikely to meet. So what do you do? You turn to the bookshops, which are flooded with a huge variety of books containing nutritional information and advice on how to cook with health as well as taste in mind. You turn to the practitioners of alternative medicine, the naturopaths, the homoeopaths, the herbalists, all those who have a working knowledge of, and interest in, sound nutrition.

Another measure of the growing awareness and importance that you, the public, place on looking after yourself is the huge mail bag which I receive at LBC. A thousand people a week write to me at the radio station. People of all ages, of both sexes, in all walks of life, even children at school – and they all have a common theme. They all want to know what they can do to help themselves with a particular health problem, what they can do to help themselves remain fit, vital and active. They don't want panaceas, they don't want pills; they want self-help and that, I think, is the fundamental difference between alternative and orthodox medicine. Doctors discourage patients from involvement in their own treatment. The alternative practitioners not only encourage the patients to be involved in their own care, but many of them insist on self-help as the first vital step on the long road to optimum health.

Alternative or complementary

There is no such thing as alternative medicine. There is good medicine and there is bad medicine and this is true on both sides of the dividing line between orthodox and unorthodox practices. Not so long ago many patients who came to me were afraid to tell their general practitioner because they felt that he would have nothing further to do with them if they visited an osteopath. This was certainly true in many cases. Today, however, attitudes have changed considerably. Doctors are allowed to refer their patients to practitioners of the unorthodox forms of therapy without fear of being struck off the medical register.

There are still many doctors who resent the intrusion of the complementary practitioners into what they regard as their own private world of healing the sick. In fairness, I am bound to say that there are many practitioners of the alternative therapies who in turn are totally dismissive of modern scientific interventive medicine. These are the practitioners who say that no patient should ever take a drug if it is not a herb or homoeopathic. These are the practitioners who say that there is never a need to resort to surgery. One wonders how they would react if their child contracted a life-threatening severe infectious disease. Would they allow the child to take antibiotics? What would they do if their child developed acute appendicitis? Would they leave the appendix where it was to rupture and possibly cause peritonitis or death? I think not. The excesses of this type of practitioner do far more harm than good to the cause of natural therapeutics.

Of course, there are many doctors who are highly sceptical of the claims of alternative practitioners, but it is up to every one of us involved in the professions to bridge the gap that stands between us. We have to communicate with the doctors. We have to explain to them what we are doing and why we are doing it. We have to convince them that we are serious about our work and that we are not quacks and charlatans cashing in on what is currently a popular craze in our country.

One of the many benefits which I gained from compiling and presenting the weekly Body Talk programme is that I have had the opportunity to meet and talk to a wide range of people, including

11

physicians, surgeons, pathologists and GPs from every field of orthodox medicine. In a recent interview with a consultant orthopaedic surgeon from Stoke Mandeville Hospital I asked his opinion of osteopathy. His reply was, 'I think that osteopaths have a very valuable part to play in the treatment of low back pain.' He went on to say that he frequently referred his patients to an osteopath. These were the patients whose back problem did not justify the consideration of invasive surgery and who he felt would not respond well to the normal orthodox treatments of back pain, especially plaster corsets, bed rest, traction or physiotherapy. I went on to ask how he chose which osteopath to refer his patients to and his answer was very simple. 'I send my patients,' he said, 'to the osteopaths who send their patients to me.' He went on to say that by this he meant any osteopath who knew when the patient's condition did not warrant manipulative treatment but was of a more serious nature and could well end in surgery, and that osteopath then took the appropriate steps to see that the patient was properly investigated by a surgeon. He said he would be happy to work with any osteopath who showed this degree of skill, knowledge and responsibility.

An eminent cancer surgeon working with the Marie Curie Foundation told me that he was in great sympathy with the nutritional ideas of the naturopaths. Furthermore, he was firmly convinced that food played a vital role not only in the causation of many cancers but also in treatment. He was in favour of the type of nutritional approach being adopted by institutions such as the Bristol Cancer Clinic.

A leading consultant psychiatrist of one of the London teaching hospitals said on the Body Talk programme that he was interested in 'healing' as a form of treatment and was in no way against seeing it practised within the framework of the National Health Service. So you see, not all doctors are anti alternative therapists.

A recent survey of 86 recently qualified doctors, all GPs, found that 76 of them believed acupuncture to be useful, 74 of them believed in hypnosis, 45 thought that homoeopathy was useful and 39 of them that osteopathy had a part to play in medical treatments. Eighteen of these doctors were themselves treating patients with one or more of the alternative therapies and over a third of them had already referred some of their patients to alternative practitioners. Twenty-two of these young doctors had already themselves received treatment from an alternative therapist and 80 per cent of them said that they would like to learn at least one of the alternative therapies as an adjunct to their medical practice.

Throughout the orthodox medical world, from the highest pinnacles of medical achievement to the youngest undergraduate medical student taking the first faltering steps up the ladder of his chosen career, there is a groundswell of interest in alternatives and of dissatisfaction with some aspects of modern technological medicine. During an interview a GP said to me that one of the reasons for the massive overprescribing of drugs in this country, especially of tranquillisers, was that writing the prescription was without doubt the quickest way of terminating the consultation.

In some ways modern medicine has lost its sense of direction. I believe that more and more orthodox doctors want to turn the clock back a little. This is not to deny the wonderful advances in surgical techniques and the development of many life-saving drugs, but to go back to an era when there was time for the bedside manner, when doctors were trained to care for people. I think that because of these feelings, doctors are looking closely at alternative therapies.

For this very reason it is vital that the alternative practitioners set out to carry their message to those still unconvinced of the efficacy of some of our therapies. But we must all accept the fact that we need each other and by all I don't mean just the practitioners, both medical and alternative, but patients too. There are things that we do better than the doctors. There are things that we do as well as the doctors. There are things that we cannot do. Likewise, for the orthodox doctors, there are many areas in which we could help them to help their patients. And, after all, in the end the only thing that really matters in any form of healing is that the patient receives the best treatment for his condition and that this treatment is administered with care, love, consideration and, above all, dignity. It is for this reason that I am convinced that alternative medicine is not the right word.

Complementary medicine implies a situation where in the care of any patient, any problem, a variety of different therapists can use their different skills and different methods of treatment in ways which complement each other to the benefit of the suffering patient. There are practitioners on the unorthodox side of the fence who believe that complementary means subordinate. This is not true. Nobody is suggesting these therapies should be supplementary or under the control of any other practitioners, but if we all work together for the benefit of humanity, how much pain could be avoided. How much unnecessary disease could be forestalled. How much money could be saved in the Health Service by reducing the horrendous drugs bill, by minimising the amount of unnecessary surgery and by freeing beds and scarce resources for the treatment of conditions for which they are both warranted and designed.

The therapies: what, how and when

The purpose of this book is to enable readers to find for themselves the type of therapy which would best suit any particular problem from which they might be suffering. So we need to take a look at the most important of the complementary therapies – what they are, how they work and when they are appropriate in the treatment of disease. We shall look at acupuncture, naturopathy, osteopathy, herbalism and homoeopathy. But first a few words to the wise.

The practice of orthodox medicine in this country is strictly controlled by legislation. Any doctor who misbehaves either personally or professionally is liable to have his name removed from the Register of the General Medical Council. This to all intents and purposes prevents him from practising his profession in this country. Sadly, there is no such legal statutory register for practitioners of complementary medicine. Several attempts have been made to establish such a register but they have all fallen by the wayside over the years.

If you are considering visiting a practitioner of complementary medicine, check up on his qualifications. There are a number of professional bodies in this country who do publish professional registers of their members and these registers imply basic levels of training, competence, professional conduct and, most importantly, insurance. Do not be impressed by long rows of important-sounding letters after the practitioner's name. There are lists of professional qualifications that do have some meaning. The most important thing is that the practitioner should belong to one of the reputable bodies and you will find a list of those at the end of the book. Titles, qualifications and impressive credentials can all be bogus. They are just as easy to obtain from mail order correspondence courses, short weekends arranged by bogus colleges, schools and other establishments, or they can be totally self-awarded and figments of the practitioner's fertile imagination.

There seems to be a concept that complementary medicine, because it is natural, is safe. Sadly, that is not true. There are many herbs, for instance, which are highly toxic; in fact any medicament, natural or synthetic, that has a therapeutic effect is liable to have a side effect. In the same way, acupuncture in the wrong hands can be a serious hazard to health. One has to look at the question of sterility of needles, apart from whether the practitioner knows where he's putting them. Manipulative skills in the right hands can be a boon to the suffering patient. In the wrong hands they can spell disaster. The competent practitioner has to be capable of two things: he has to be able to make a correct diagnosis of the patient's problem and he has to be competent in the practice of the particular therapeutic skills which he uses.

There is no doubt that a vast majority of reputable practitioners in the field of complementary medicine are highly skilled and highly trained, but as the orthopaedic surgeon said earlier in the book, the osteopath who knows when not to treat the patient is far more impressive than the osteopath who treats every patient for every condition. For this reason, and for this reason alone, a sound background training in conventional medicine and diagnostic skills is vital if the practitioner is to be safe to practise on the public. Any school which is not teaching its would-be practitioners anatomy, physiology and differential diagnosis and is not exposing those students to a larger volume of patient material which he can observe and treat under supervision is doing a grave disservice not only to the public at large but also to its own chosen profession.

Acupuncture and traditional Chinese medicine

The origins of Chinese traditional medicine are shrouded in the mists of antiquity. Acupuncture, the treatment which involves the piercing of the skin with a needle, is certainly the most well-known aspect of Chinese medicine in the Western world, although it forms only a part of the concept. Traditional Chinese medicine includes the use of many thousands of herbs, diet, nutrition, manipulation, massage and exercise, both physical and spiritual. The earliest writings on acupuncture date back some 4500 years and Chinese folklore tells how doctors tending ancient Chinese warriors noticed many reports of soldiers recovering from chronic illnesses after receiving stab or arrow wounds during battle. It became apparent that the size of the wound mattered very little, but the location and the depth of penetration were vitally important. From these early observations, the Chinese developed an entire system of acupuncture.

How acupuncture works

The basic concepts of acupuncture are fundamentally very simple. The ancient Chinese believed that human life, in fact all life, was sustained by a flow of vital energy or life force known as Chi and that this force was made up of two exactly equal and opposite components, Yin and Yang. The object of using acupuncture was to balance the relative levels of Yin and Yang, thus maintaining a balanced flow of Chi throughout the entire system of the body, throughout the organs, nerves, the brain, the skin, the respiratory system.

This balance was equated with good health. With the advent of illness, disturbances of this flow of energy were noticed and the detection of the disturbances relied upon the traditional Chinese method of pulse diagnosis, wherein the practitioner felt the twelve pulses, six in each wrist, which relate to the specific lines of flow of the energy. These lines are known as meridians. They are arbitrary lines on the body's surface upon which lie the key acupuncture points. There are twenty-six of these meridians containing in all some 800 recognised points, and needles can be inserted into the skin at the precise point required to achieve either stimulation or sedation, to increase or reduce levels of energy flowing through that point and thus into meridians.

Today most acupuncturists use needles made of stainless steel, though in earliest times the Chinese used needles made of stone, bamboo, bone and finally metal, when they were sometimes made from precious metals such as silver, gold or even alloys. The Western acupuncturist will probably combine a mixture of the best of the traditional approaches of Chinese medicine with the diagnostic skills and techniques available to modern medicine. A basic diagnosis will still rely on the pulses, and the acupuncturist will then decide which points need to be treated in order to achieve the stability of Chi energy.

The acupuncturist may choose to carry out this treatment by the insertion of needles, which in the right hands is a perfectly safe and usually painless procedure. He may choose to use heat, in a system called moxibustion, in which the dried leaves of the herb *Artemisia vulgaris* are used to heat the surface of the skin over the acupuncture point. A more intense method of treatment is to wrap a small plug of the herb around the already inserted acupuncture needle, thus transferring the heat of the burning herb through the needle, through the acupuncture point and into the meridian being treated.

The influence of modern Western science on the practice of acupuncture has been profound. The discovery that certain acupuncture points trigger the release of chemicals in the brain known as endorphins and enkephalins has helped to convince the sceptical Western scientists that acupuncture as a therapy has real value. These chemicals act in the same way as morphine on the body's nervous system, and this would explain why the use of acupuncture in anaesthesia has been so successful. Many major operations are performed daily in China using acupuncture needles as the only form of anaesthetic.

The advantages of this system are obvious. It relieves the patient of the shock of anaesthesia, and it enables patients who could not otherwise stand conventional gas anaesthetics, due to respiratory or cardiac problems, to undergo surgery far more safely. The patients recover immediately the operation is completed and Western observers have seen patients rise from the operating table and leave the theatre unaided. The development of electro-acupuncture is an instance of the combination of Western science with traditional Chinese philosophy. Small electronic machines are now available which can actually detect the acupuncture point on the skin and furthermore can measure the amount of Chi energy flowing through the point. Electrical impulses can be used to stimulate the point and the machine can measure the amount of energy either being used to stimulate or withdrawn from the system to sedate a particular meridian.

Sadly, one of the side effects of this involvement of science in acupuncture is that many Western practitioners believe that acupuncture is only of proven value as a treatment for the relief of pain. They believe this because these effects can be demonstrated and measured in a laboratory. The traditional acupuncturist, however, knows from personal experience that the value of acupuncture goes far further than mere analgesia. The practitioner who is skilled and trained can use his art, for it surely is an art more than a science, to treat patients suffering from the whole range of diseases.

In traditional Chinese medicine there are no names for diseases, because the traditional practitioner only treats people, not symptoms. The Chinese, too, were the earliest pioneers of preventative medicine, and folklore tells us that the traditional Chinese physician visited his patients regularly to ensure that they were well. As long as they were, he received payment. As soon as a patient fell ill, payment stopped and the patient would not pay again until restored to health. One can't help wondering what the application of this concept would do to the exclusive private practices of Harley Street.

Visiting the acupuncturist

First make sure that your acupuncturist is a member of one of the recognised bodies and don't be afraid to check up on his or her qualifications when making the appointment. On arrival at the surgery, have a look around and see if it's clean and hygienic. After all, acupuncture involves piercing the skin with needles and this is a potential source of infection and disease if not carried out in hygienic conditions. Is the acupuncturist clean? Are his fingernails clean? Are there obviously facilities for sterilisation of his needles? On your first visit the acupuncturist will probably take a normal case history as you would expect from any medical practitioner. If he doesn't, ask him why not. He will then probably proceed to feel the pulses in your wrists. This might take some considerable time. He will then decide how best to treat you and your particular problem.

If you are in acute pain, it is likely that you will be treated with what are known as secondary doctor techniques, that is needles applied to or near the site of pain in order to give you rapid relief from the discomfort. This is not the general practice in the relief of the cause of your problem, merely a local treatment to stop the pain. Needles will be inserted into the skin and may well be left there for anything between ten and twenty minutes, during which time the needles can be stimulated by rotation or gentle agitation up and down.

In the treatment of systemic complaints the area treated may well seem far removed from the site of your problem. For instance, migraine may be treated by inserting needles into the feet, digestive problems by treating the points in the hands. Reference to the diagrams (see list of illustrations on page vii) will show you which meridians relate to which organs and functions of the body. Most patients say that they feel an amazing sense of relaxation within a few seconds of the needles being inserted. There are of course dangers in any form of therapy and acupuncture is not without them. The most serious problem is that of transmitting blood diseases, especially hepatitis. The hepatitis virus cannot usually be destroyed simply by boiling, so all reputable acupuncturists use some more sophisticated form of sterilisation. Furthermore, the patients should be asked if they have ever suffered from hepatitis and those patients should have a set of needles used exclusively for them. When the patient's course of treatment is complete, these needles should be safely disposed of. The additional hazard of AIDS must also be considered, and the practitioner must be aware of factors that make this awful illness a likely problem.

The other possible danger with acupuncture treatment is that of damaging underlying organs. Naturally, treatment of the arms, legs and extremities is comparatively safe, but when treating the abdomen, chest, neck or head, the acupuncturist must always be conscious of the tissues and organs that lie beneath the area that he is treating. There have been reported cases of serious injury inflicted by the careless use of acupuncture needles. One of the most famous of these cases was, interestingly enough, when a consultant hospital surgeon who had done a weekend course of acupuncture succeeded in puncturing the lung of his patient with an acupuncture needle. This doctor was severely reprimanded and the patient compensated.

Sometimes in the day or two following acupuncture treatment, especially when stimulation rather than sedation is involved, patients do report fairly strong reactions to the treatment. These normally subside within forty-eight hours and leave the patient feeling considerably more comfortable.

It takes many years to learn the skills and techniques of acupuncture. In the right hands it is a safe, highly effective and useful therapy in the treatment of many health problems and you can safely entrust your health care to a properly trained and registered acupuncturist.

When to visit an acupuncturist

The traditional concept of Chinese medicine is that it is a complete system of healing. Few acupuncturists in the world, however, embrace all aspects of Chinese medicine. Nonetheless, the range of problems which respond well to acupuncture is large and impressive. Physical conditions for which pain is the major symptom are extremely well treated with acupuncture. Joint diseases such as arthritis, rheumatoid arthritis, muscular problems, lumbago, sciatica, disc problems, trigeminal neuralgia and post-operative pain are just some of the areas where acupuncture as an analgesic is extremely effective. Chronic problems like migraine, asthma, hay fever, chronic rhinitis and skin problems like eczema, psoriasis and acne all respond to acupuncture, though of course the results are better when this treatment is used in conjunction with other natural therapies.

Acupuncture can also be used most successfully in the treatment of liver, kidney and bowel disorders, particularly those of the digestive system such as irritable bowel syndrome, Crohn's disease, diverticulitis, colitis, chronic constipation and gall bladder problems, though once again these are best treated in combination with other therapies such as herbal medicines and naturopathic nutrition.

Acupuncture has proved to be extremely effective in dealing with addictive problems: addiction to sleeping pills, tranquillisers, illicit drugs, tobacco and alcohol can all be treated successfully. The techniques vary. Some practitioners use needles inserted into the ear which remain *in situ*. Others prefer the patient to come regularly for treatments in which the needles are inserted during the treatment and removed before the patient leaves. The best results have been achieved with smoking and hard drug addiction. In my experience the treatment of alcoholics has not been so successful, although this is of course far more of a social problem than a purely medical one.

As with the treatment of all addictive problems, the entire success of the procedure depends first and foremost on the patient's desire and motivation to give up the habit to which he is addicted. Without the patient's co-operation, little can be achieved. However, in my own practice, we achieve an average 70 per cent success rate with people who *want* to give up smoking and long-term results also seem to be equally encouraging, in that the majority of those who succeed are still non-smokers two to three years after their initial course of treatment. At times of stress, it is useful for the patient to have one or two booster treatments which seem to make the difference between continued success or a dismal return to the old habits. How much these boosters work through reinforcement of the patient's psychological desire not to smoke again or through the physiological effects of the acupuncture I do not really understand, but the end definitely justifies the means.

Naturopathy

Naturopathy, or nature cure as it is sometimes known, is without doubt the great-grandfather of many of the other branches of alternative medicine. The underlying philosophies of nature cure have spread their tentacles into the structures of therapies such as osteopathy, chiropractic, homoeopathy and herbal medicine, and whilst these may differ greatly in technical application, they all use the founding principles of naturopathy as a starting point for the practice of their special therapies.

Despite the fact that the word naturopathy was not used until the beginning of this century, the philosophical basis and many of the methods of naturopathic medicine are ancient, dating back to about 400 BC when Hippocrates first propounded his philosophical basis for the treatment of disease. Here was the first explanation of the treatment of illness by harnessing nature's laws. It is very strange that although Hippocrates is dubbed the father of medicine, modern medical science completely ignores the more than self-evident laws of health which were laid down by him nearly 2500 years ago. It was he who said that only nature heals, provided it is given the opportunity to do so. Disease, he stated, is an expression of purification. And finally, his concept that all disease is one showed an insight and an intuitive knowledge of the innermost workings of the human organs that was centuries in advance of his time.

The philosophy of naturopathy is based on three basic principles. First, the body possesses the power to heal itself through its own internal vitality. Harnessing this vital force is the cornerstone of naturopathic philosophy. All naturopathic treatments aim at increasing, enhancing and mobilising the body's own innate defence and repair mechanisms, whilst at the same time doing nothing which might interfere with those mechanisms.

Secondly, the naturopath believes that disease is always a manifestation of the vital forms of the body being used to remove obstruction to normal function. A naturopathic practitioner seeks to discover and remove the basic causes of disease and not merely to treat the symptoms. For example, chemical disturbance of the body can be due to dietary deficiencies or excesses. They can be due to a malfunction of the eliminative processes. They can be related to inefficient circulation or disturbances of the breathing. Mechanical problems can be caused by muscular tension, damaged ligaments or joints, poor posture, especially that due to occupational factors, as well as to spinal misalignments which lead to an interference with the functioning of the nervous system and of the musculo-skeletal system in general. Finally, impairment of the psychological function can be produced by stress, caused by worry, tension, anxiety in personal, domestic and work situations.

Thirdly, the principle that naturopathic medicine is holistic is essential to the sound application of naturopathic methods. Disease affects the entire organism, not simply an isolated system or organ. Every human being responds in an individual way to his or her environment. Each has separate strengths and weaknesses. Each has separate needs. Their body's reactions to the same stress may be very different depending on health, genetic tendencies or previous history.

In treating the whole person, the naturopath searches for the cause at many levels. He attempts to eliminate the fundamental cause of illness and does not simply try to remove the symptoms of disease. To the sedentary office worker, an ingrowing toenail is a painful but not disastrous inconvenience. To the professional ballet dancer an ingrowing toenail can spell the ruination of their career. Whilst technically the treatment of both toenails would be the same, the psychological and emotional response of the two patients would be totally different. The mechanical treatment of both toenails would naturally be the same, but whereas the office worker needs advice on the type of shoes or socks he is wearing and guidance as to ways of avoiding recurrence of the problem, the ballet dancer needs a far greater level of emotional support and reassurance since anything which affects a dancer's feet quite understandably produces psycho-emotional responses of fear, anxiety and enormous stress.

The true naturopath fulfils a dual role. First, patients consult him with a particular problem so that his therapeutic skills can be used to resolve the underlying causes of the complaint with which the patient presents him. Secondly, and more importantly, he fulfils the role of an educator. It is the responsibility of the naturopath to educate his patient to take more responsibility for his own health; to assist him in the understanding of the fundamental laws of nature relating to rest, exercise and nutrition; and to guide him towards a lifestyle which, while still appropriate for today's society, will help the patient to avoid the excesses of our Western civilisation and consequently to lead a full, active, satisfying and above all, healthy long life.

The British Naturopathic and Osteopathic Association has listed a number of therapies which are of primary importance in naturopathic treatment for disease:

(1) *Dietetics*. This includes the prescription of balanced wholesome natural diets based on principles advocated by naturopathic practitioners for the last 100 years, and only now being accepted as correct by the orthodox medical profession and nutritionists. Also, specific controlled diets may be given at the discretion

of the practitioner to patients who require a specific and probably more rigid regime for the treatment of a particular condition.

(2) *Fasting.* Controlled fasting has been used as a form of therapy for more than 2000 years. Hippocrates used it as a treatment for many diseases, since it allows the body to concentrate all its resources on dealing with disease processes rather than with the chemical process of digestion. Although the medical profession has ridiculed fasting for years, it has in recent time begun to gain a wider acceptance and its efficacy is proven in the treatment of conditions such as obesity, high blood pressure, arthritis, rheumatism, food allergies and even some psychiatric problems such as schizophrenia.

(3) *Structural adjustments.* Using osteopathy, chiropractic, neuromuscular techniques, postural re-education and remedial exercises, the naturopathic practitioner seeks to achieve a balance in the physical workings of the body, to integrate the spine, muscles, ligaments and joints of the entire organism.

(4) *Hydrotherapy.* This is the use of water both internally and externally in the form of baths, packs, compresses, sprays and douches. Hydrotherapy is of great value in many conditions and when correctly applied it can produce remarkable results in the treatment of both acute and chronic ailments.

(5) *Natural hygiene.* This includes the general care of one's body, the use of moderate and sensible physical exercise relative to the individual patient, and the cultivation of a positive approach to life and health. Relaxation techniques are an important part of this area of treatment.

(6) *Education.* In naturopathic philosophy, it is just as important, if not more so, to explain to the patient why disease occurs and what the patient can do for himself or herself to maintain the new improved level of health given to them by naturopathic approaches to treatment. In this way the patient is encouraged to take responsibility for his or her own health. Only nature heals and the naturopath will do everything in his power to encourage that healing process inherent in the body of every single one of us. Moreover, he will do nothing which interferes with that healing process.

When do you go to the naturopath?

Most naturopathic practices are similar in concept to the general practice of orthodox medicine. Most people, once they discover naturopathy for themselves, tend to use their naturopath as their family health adviser. A properly trained naturopath will take a normal medical history on your first visit, but will also be far more interested in your lifestyle than the average medical practitioner.

He will want to know about your eating habits, your working habits, your sleeping habits, your general emotional state, your sense of fulfilment, your frustrations, your angers, your fears, as well as being concerned with the normal physiological functions such as blood tests, urine tests and blood pressure.

There is hardly a medical condition which will not benefit from naturopathic treatment. It may often happen that the naturopath will recognise the need for therapies beyond his normal range of practice in your particular case. It may be, for example, that you require surgery. A naturopath does not give up at this point. He will try to ensure that when you have had his treatment it will complement that of the surgeon whom you are about to visit. He will improve your nutrition. He may prescribe vitamin therapy. In short, he will do everything to ensure that you are in the optimum state of health to undergo the surgery and to recover from it as quickly as is possible.

Osteopathy

'It is necessary to know the nature of the spine, what its natural purposes are, for such a knowledge will be requisite for many diseases.' This quote from Hippocrates was written in 400 BC. What is osteopathy? Osteopathy is a system of healing that deals with the structure of the body, that is the bones, joints, ligaments, tendons, muscles and general connecting tissue and their relationship with one another.

The term osteopathy was first used by its founder, Dr Andrew Taylor Still, in 1874 to describe a philosophy for the practice of healing that he had developed himself. He believed that the human body was self-healing and that an uninterrupted nerve and blood supply to all tissues of the body was indispensable to their normal function. If any structural problems, muscle spasm, curvature of the spine or injury interfered with this nerve and blood flow, the self-healing power was interfered with and disease would result. With this in mind he devised a system of manipulation intended to realign any structural deviations and abnormalities.

Still was the first person to put forward any rational explanation as to why the spine was so important in the maintenance of health, enclosing as it does the spinal cord. The spinal cord can be described as an extension of the brain which controls all the functions of the body, not only muscles, but also tissues such as the vital organs, heart, liver, lungs, kidneys, blood vessels and veins. Any interference with the nerves passing to and from the brain via the spinal cord must affect the normal functions of the tissues to which those nerves are connected.

Manipulation itself has a long history. Hippocrates described various techniques for treating the spine more than 2000 years ago, whilst many primitive yet effective forms of manipulation still exist in folk medicine all over the world. However, its use up to this time is purely in the treatment of conditions of the back. What Still did was to extend the use of manipulation to cover the treatment of a whole host of other conditions where impaired structure affected function. He was able to adopt many of those techniques which were valuable and reject those which were of no use or possibly even dangerous, thus creating new techniques in order to have a complete and practical therapy at his disposal.

What do osteopaths treat?

Most people first consult an osteopath complaining of back problems or, nearly as often, of pain and discomfort in other joints and muscles. However, it is not unusual to find that after treatment for the chief complaint, patients also report improvement in other conditions from which they may be suffering and which they did not consider worth bringing to the osteopath's attention. For example, a patient suffering from neck and shoulder stiffness and pain may find that manipulation of the neck has also relieved dizziness. Experiences such as these lend support to Still's concept that spinal problems can and do affect not only muscles and joints, but also other tissues and organs that receive the nerve supply from the problem area.

Modern research in American osteopathic hospitals has shown how abnormalities of the spinal cord can affect organs such as the lungs, heart, stomach, intestines, bladder, uterus and so on. It can also be proved that these organs are able to affect the spinal cord. Manipulation of the spine, therefore, can be shown to be of great value in the treatment of many organic conditions, especially migraine, asthma, constipation, period pains, heart disease and digestive disorders.

Osteopathy does not, however, consider the spine to be the only factor in disease. It cannot deny that genetic development, dietary, environmental, psychological and bacterial factors also cause disease, nor can it claim to cure diseases brought about by these factors.

What does osteopathic treatment involve?

Before an osteopath treats a patient, he takes a detailed medical history. This is followed by a complete physical examination. He will examine the patient's posture, the way in which he moves, plus observing restrictions or exaggerations of movement in any area. The osteopath makes a detailed examination of the spine, testing the movement of each vertebra, looking for tenderness, stiffness or displacement. If necessary, he may also recommend further tests such as X-rays or blood or urine tests to help him reach an exact diagnosis. Having made his diagnosis and established the cause of the condition, the osteopath will begin treatment, assuming that it is both advisable and safe to do so. The purpose of treatment is to improve the mobility of impaired joints, to restore functions to joints which are not working properly and to relieve areas of pressure which may be affecting nerves often supplying very distant parts of the body.

The osteopath may use techniques of manipulation, deep neuro-muscular massage, relaxation and postural re-education, all with the object of relieving the cause of the patient's condition.

It is not abnormal for patients to suffer some form of reaction after the first one or two osteopathic treatments, since the high velocity thrust used to readjust the spinal joints can sometimes irritate surrounding tissues. Patients often expect the osteopath not to be in favour of the use of drugs or surgery for the treatment of back problems and this in broad principle is true, although there are situations when anti-inflammatory drugs or painkillers can be recommended in times of acute pain. As for surgery, there are situations in which spinal surgery is inevitable. Most osteopaths, however, believe that many patients submit to surgery before exploring all the alternative possibilities of manipulative treatment. There is no doubt that more and more orthopaedic surgeons are recommending their patients to try osteopathic treatment where other orthodox forms have failed before resorting to spinal surgery. The complementary use of the skills of the orthodox orthopaedic surgeon and the osteopath is surely in the best interest of the patient and produces results which in some instances neither practitioner could achieve on his own.

Yet again, it is the holistic approach of the osteopath which is the fundamental reason for the enormous success osteopaths achieve in the treatment of back problems. The number of patients who have suffered back problems for years and have never been examined properly by any orthodox medical practitioner is quite staggering. The osteopath will look at the patient as a whole entity. Although back pain may be the symptom with which the patient presents himself in the osteopath's surgery, the root cause of that pain can be very far removed from the back itself. There are a number of medical problems which do cause pain in the back, but there are also many more simple, practical abnormalities or difficulties which can result in back ache.

The osteopath's examination of the patient begins from the moment he enters the consulting room door. How does he walk, how is his posture, how are his movements, is he stiff and rigid, is he bent at the waist, is his back out of alignment? How does he sit in the chair? All these things are vital clues to the origin of the patient's problem. Many patients who have repeatedly visited their doctor with back ache have never been asked to take their clothes off. No osteopathic examination is complete without a full examination of the patient so that the practitioner can inspect the posture with the patient standing, sitting and lying without clothes on.

It is quite remarkable how frequently simple problems with the feet, ankles, knees or hips can result in back pain; how frequently changing the chair in which the patient works, altering the height of a bench in the factory or workshop, or merely changing the type of shoes which the patient wears can dramatically improve long-lasting and chronic back problems.

There are several thousand practitioners in this country who title themselves osteopaths. However, a mere 1000 of these belong to the organised and responsible professional bodies whose requisites for membership are completion of a four-year full-time course of training. A list of associations appears at the back of the book (page 287).

Chiropractic

Chiropractic is another form of manipulative treatment closely allied to osteopathy. A concept of chiropractic was developed by David Daniel Palmer in 1895 in the state of Iowa in America. He believed, like Still, that displacements of the structure of the spine caused pressure on nerves which in turn caused symptoms in distant parts of the body. The main differences between chiropractic and osteopathy are mostly historical, since both forms of manipulative therapy now subscribe to modern concepts of anatomy and physiology, although they both use manipulative treatment for the relief of a wide range of disorders, not just disorders of the spine.

Chiropractic tends to place greater reliance on X-rays in the diagnosis of spinal problems, and the actual techniques of manipulation are slightly different from those of the osteopath, the chiropractor tending to use less leverage and more direct thrust against specific vertebrae.

Properly qualified chiropractors are highly trained professionals and achieve excellent results in the treatment of back pain and other musculo-skeletal disorders. Chiropractic is more widespread in America and other parts of the world, although the establishment of the Anglo-European College of Chiropractic in Bournemouth has greatly increased the numbers of qualified practising chiropractors in the United Kingdom.

Herbal medicine

The use of plants to relieve human suffering is as ancient as man himself. The Chinese kept detailed written lists of herbal remedies more than 5000 years ago. The Ebers Papyrus dating from about 1500 BC contained detailed descriptions of the preparation of herbal and other remedies. Many of these remedies are certain to have been effective. We know that many of the plants used contained powerful chemicals which have active effects on the physiology of the human body. One specific prescription in the Ebers Papyrus was for the treatment of night blindness and for this it was recommended to take the liver of an ox, to roast it, to crush it to a paste and feed it to the patient who was suffering from night blindness. We know today that this prescription must have been effective, because roasted ox liver contains large quantities of vitamin A. There are scientific validations for many of the traditional herbal remedies.

The great physician Paracelsus did much to formalise the written knowledge of herbal medicines and he was followed in England by the great herbalists Culpeper and Hill. In fact Culpeper's book *The English Physician and Complete Herbal*, which was published in 1653, was one of the first medical texts to be written in English rather than Latin. Culpeper did not make many friends amongst the medical profession for translating their secrets into a language understood by the common man.

A medicinal plant can be any type of plant which provides material of therapeutic activity. This material can be derived from the root, the rhizome, stem, leaf, flower, seed, bark, fruits, woods, gums or resins which are collected from the plant. Whilst some Western scientists mock the usefulness of herbal medicines, one does not need to look far to discover that many of the synthetic preparations manufactured by the huge pharmaceutical industries owe their origins to discoveries of the great medical herbalists. Atropine and other associated alkaloids are derived from deadly nightshade. Ergometrine and ergotamine come from the ergot plant. Cocaine comes from the coca plant. The humble garden foxglove yields digitalis, whilst morphine is derived from the opium poppy and the yam is a source of hormones for the manufacture of the contraceptive pill. These few examples serve to illustrate the wide range of clinical effects that can be produced by herbal medicines. The ones mentioned are of course amongst the most powerful, but there are many, many hundreds of other useful, safe and effective plants, medicines derived from which are prescribed with great benefit and effect by the trained herbalist.

It is interesting that in other parts of the world, specifically in Eastern Europe, there are state-run herbal pharmacies and it is to these that patients turn first when they are unwell. They act as a primary care centre, the herbalist offering simple, safe and effective treatment for many minor ailments and preventing patients taking up valuable time with the doctor in his surgery for complaints which can be treated so easily. Moreover, potential harmful side-effects of simple herbal remedies are far less toxic and far less insidious than those of many of the modern drugs.

The herbalist prepares his remedies in a number of different ways. The most powerful remedies are made up as tinctures in which one part of the herb is saturated in five parts of alcohol. Liquid extracts which contain one part by weight of the herb in one part by volume of the extract are also often used. Herbs can be used as infusions. These are usually made from the exposed part of the plant (flowers, leaves, stems or sometimes all three), as opposed to being made from the roots. A teaspoon of the dried herb is placed in a cupful of just boiling water and is covered and left to stand for at least ten minutes. The more woody parts of the plant are used to make a decoction where the roots, twigs, berries, bark or seeds can be used. These are put into a saucepan with cold water and brought to a boil. The pan is simmered for twenty to thirty minutes. This extracts all the active ingredients from the plant's constituents.

The value of the poultice has been sadly neglected by many practitioners, both orthodox and alternative, in recent years. However, farmers and veterinary surgeons know better. They continue to use poultices to great effect. The poultice works on the basis of the volatile oils of the plant penetrating the skin of an affected area. Poultices are extremely effective in dealing with the problems of abcesses and other local inflammations. Powdered comfrey root, slippery elm bark or marshmallow root are the most frequently used. The poultice is made by mixing a tablespoon of the powdered herb moistened with hot water into a thick paste. It is also sometimes prepared by using herbal tea such as comfrey or camomile. The paste is then smeared on to pieces of clean lint, folded into another piece of clean lint and applied to the inflamed area as hot as the patient can stand.

Compresses are another extremely valuable form of treatment with herbal remedies. Compresses made with tincture of arnica can be very effective in the relief of sprains, strains and severe bruising. Ointments can also be made with herbal extracts using beeswax to create the required consistency. Extremely useful ointments are calendula (marigold) and marshmallow, both of which are very effective in the relief of scratches, burns, insect bites and other minor skin irritations.

Herbal medicines lend themselves well to simple self-medication and first-aid procedures for minor complaints. However, the extreme potency and wide range of efficacy of many herbal remedies has led to the growth of a thriving profession of practising herbalists. In this country the National Institute of Medical Herbalists of Great Britain was founded in 1864 and runs its own training college, graduates of which are entitled to join the register and become members of the National Institute of Medical Herbalists.

Mounting anxiety over the side-effects of drugs and the repeated publicity given to drug disasters has led to a boom in the practice of herbal medicine. More and more members of the public are anxious to avoid the possible dangers of drug therapy when there are simpler, effective measures that can be taken. Parents too are increasingly anxious about their children receiving repeated doses of antibiotics, painkillers and other over-prescribed medicines.

The qualified herbalist will treat his patient in the same way as any other professional in the Health Service. He will need a full history of your medical background. He will, however, be equally interested in your state of nutrition and your general lifestyle and, in common with all holistic practitioners, will not merely be interested in helping to relieve your symptoms without delving into the cause of the disease.

Homoeopathy

Similia similibus curantur/Like is healed by like

This was the theory published in 1796 of the origins of homoeopathy. Its founder, Samuel Christian Hahnemann, was born in Meissen in Germany in 1745 and having studied medicine at Leipzig and Vienna, he settled down in Leipzig to follow his career. During his researches he came across a well-known but uninvestigated fact and this was that the symptoms produced by quinine in a healthy body were remarkably similar to the symptoms which quinine was used to treat. Hahnemann devoted the rest of his life to studying the possibilities of curing like with like. He also developed the system of potentisation, that is of using smaller and smaller doses of a particular drug to produce more and more powerful effects.

In spite of tremendous antagonism from his rivals in medicine and being forced to leave Leipzig, Hahnemann created a system of medicine which has spread throughout the world and is widely used wherever medicine is practised. The basic concept of Hahnemann's view of medicine was that disease did not exist as a separate entity. He believed that disease was 'an aberration from the state of health' and his work revolved around finding homoeopathic remedies which reproduced the symptoms of every possible variation of these aberrations from the state of health.

Homoeopathy is unique amongst the alternative therapies for two reasons. Firstly, it is available under the Health Service and there are a number of homoeopathic hospitals in this country. Secondly, homoeopathic medicine enjoys official royal patronage. This state of affairs resulted from the original introduction of homoeopathy to England by Frederick Quinn, a young English doctor with the highest social connections. In fact he is rumoured to have been an illegitimate son of the Duchess of Devonshire. The orthodox practitioners in England were no more enamoured of Quinn than Hahnemann's contemporaries were of him in Leipzig, but through his connections Quinn made homoeopathy a firm favourite with the Royal Family and many other eminent people. For this reason homoeopathy enjoys the status in England that it does today. The centre of British homoeopathic activity is the Royal London Homoeopathic Hospital together with its faculty of homoeopathic medicine. In spite of royal connections and a superb hospital, the general interest amongst orthodox medical practitioners is not only very slight, but their knowledge of even the basic concepts of homoeopathy is negligible.

There is also in this country a large body of non-medical homoeopaths. The differences between the medically trained and other homoeopaths are not as great as one might think, since both schools follow the four basic rules which have evolved from Hahnemann's original teachings. First, homoeopathic medicines should be chosen because of the similarity between the symptoms which they produce in a normal person and the symptoms from which the patient is suffering. Secondly, medicine should wherever possible be given singly. Thirdly, the medicines are given in small homoeopathic doses. Fourthly, patients should not take repeated routine doses of medication, and the medicines should only be used when the symptoms demand it.

Preparation of homoeopathic remedies

Most homoeopathic medicines are prepared from fresh material, either from plant, animal or other biological sources. The plant material is made into a tincture by being dissolved in pure alcohol. The mother tincture is then used to prepare the homoeopathic remedy. This is done by taking one drop of the tincture and mixing it with 99 drops of alcohol. It is then diluted and shaken in a special machine which Hahnemann believed imbued the medicine with a particular energy. One drop of the resulting solution is mixed again with a further 99 drops and so on and so on. The more times the process is repeated, the weaker the dilution of the original substance and, according to homoeopathic theory, the higher the potency or effectiveness of the medicine. Homoeopathic remedies are prescribed either as liquids which are taken a few drops at a time in water, or as little pilules. These are made up with inert milk sugar or sucrose as a base.

Visiting a homoeopath

Homoeopathic remedies are not prescribed in mixtures or in the broad spectrum fashion of modern pharmacological drugs. There may be dozens of remedies which would suit a patient with migraine, for instance, but there is only one remedy which will suit that individual patient with migraine. Hence the homoeopathic concept of the totality of symptoms. For this reason the homoeopathic practitioner will take an extremely detailed, lengthy case history from the patient, even going back into diseases of childhood, diseases of the parents and even possibly grandparents, as well as other close relatives.

The homoeopath will be minutely interested in things that affect the patient's condition: what makes it worse or better, how does the patient react to heat or cold? Is the patient's discomfort more on one side of the body than the other? The mere symptom of pain is of very little interest to the homoeopath, since this gives him no clue to the individuality of the patient's particular problem. The patient's psychological state is also of enormous importance to the homoeopath. What are the patient's attitudes to his own illness? Does it make him angry? Does it make him depressed? Did anything untoward happen before the onset of the illness? Was he made redundant; did he have a fight with his family; has he had a bereavement or a divorce? Has the patient suffered previous serious illnesses? Has he ever had an operation? How is the patient's complexion? What is his normal nature – easygoing, relaxed or tense, difficult and obsessive?

All these constitutional characteristics of the patient may not seem very important if you are suffering from some acute and painful condition, but to the homoeopath they are vital in arriving at the single most effective remedy for that patient at that time and with that problem. In the final analysis, the practitioner may arrive at a shortlist of five or six possible substances. It is then dependent on his own skills and intuitive feelings as to which single remedy to prescribe. The advent of modern technology has greatly simplified the prescription of homoeopathic remedies, since there are now computer programmes available which can relieve the practitioner of the time-consuming and tedious programme of cross-referencing and consulting the extensive repertories.

When to visit the homoeopath

There are a growing number of general practitioners working within the Health Service who practise homoeopathy. There are also a number of homoeopathic hospitals, including the Royal Homoeopathic Hospital in London. If you wish to be referred through the National Health Service to the Homoeopathic Hospital or a homoeopathic GP, you can ask your own doctor to give you a letter of referral. Many doctors are willing to do this, though of course there are still some sceptics who would be reluctant. However, there are also many homoeopaths who are not registered medical practitioners whom you can consult directly.

The homoeopath is a general practitioner in the truest sense of the word. Many families rely exclusively on a homoeopath for all their medical needs and the skilled practitioner will of course know when more drastic intervention is necessary in the form of surgery or other investigations. In this way, yet again, we see the advantages of a complementary system of medicine where the homoeopath, with his own particular philosophies and approaches to the patient, can work, and frequently does, in a complementary fashion with the more orthodox practitioners.

In acute conditions it may be necessary to take homoeopathic remedies two or three or even four times a day for several days. In the more long-standing chronic complaints the homoeopath may prescribe a single dose of medicament and ask you to come back to him in two weeks' time bringing a full and detailed report of what, if any, reactions have occurred since taking the single dose.

Tissue salts

During the 19th century, a German doctor named Schussler believed that disease was due to a deficiency of minerals and on this basis he developed a scheme of twelve tissue salts. These are prepared in homoeopathic concentrations and often sold in combinations. They are extremely useful for self-medication of simple ailments. The twelve tissue salts are safe, inexpensive and extremely effective remedies which are available on the shelves of every health food store and many chemists' shops.

Increasingly, orthodox scientists are demanding proof of the efficacy of any remedy and this includes homoeopathic medicines. It is extremely difficult to establish irrefutable proof of homoeopathic efficacy using the standard double blind clinical trials, since as we have already discussed, homoeopathic remedies are not prescribed on the basis of the patient's symptoms but on the basis of the patient himself. Therefore any trial which involves prescribing a specific remedy for many patients all suffering from the same symptom is bound to fail in terms of homoeopathic practice. However, homoeopathy is undoubtedly safe and undoubtedly effective for many patients.

Choosing a qualified complementary practitioner

There is a surprising boom happening in the United Kingdom. Undeterred by inflation, rising unemployment or falling pounds, there is one industry which is growing like Topsy, and with the growth come the inevitable pains, only in this industry it is you, the consumer, who are likely to end up suffering. The industry is, of course, alternative medicine, or as Prince Charles, and I, prefer to call it, complementary medicine.

All over the country natural health clinics, nutritional centres, allergy clinics, osteopaths, naturopaths, acupuncturists, reflex-ologists, chiropractors, herbalists and homoeopaths are springing up, and despite the often plush surroundings, the uniformed nurses and strings of important-sounding letters after the names, and enough certificates hanging up to look like wallpaper, these establishments may not be what they seem.

A visit to some of these places may leave you in the hands of a back street bone setter, a self-appointed nutritional counsellor, or a factory worker moonlighting as an acupuncturist after a weekend course in Wapping. Health magazines are filled with pages of advertisements for these expensive and largely useless training courses; home-study correspondence courses and week-end intensives are all on offer to anyone with the often sub-stantial funds to foot the bill and no previous experience is required.

The existence of these courses is a scandal and the so-called practitioners they turn out a danger to the public. The British College of Naturopathy and Osteopathy is the only established training centre in Europe which offers a four-year full-time course in naturopathy and osteopathy. There are only two other schools offering osteopathic training and one chiropractic college in England with the same academic entry requirements and four-year full-time courses.

The professional bodies associated with these colleges maintain registers of all qualified members and ensure proper codes of conduct and compulsory insurance for practitioners. Students from these schools are taught basic medicine and diagnostic skills and work with large numbers of patients under supervision. They are highly competent professionals, unlike the young woman patient who phoned me one afternoon to ask if she could use my steriliser as she had just completed a weekend course in acupuncture. A set of needles was included in the fee but she couldn't afford a proper machine for sterilising the needles. She had some patients coming to see her the next day.

There is no legal control over any practitioner of complementary medicine, no official register, no checks of hygiene or competence. Anyone can set up in practice with little or no training.

None of the long-established bodies in complementary medicine allows uncontrolled advertising, so avoid those that claim cures. The chances are that their qualifications are questionable. Don't be afraid to ask questions about practitioners' training. Be suspicious of evasive and belligerent answers.

As the medical profession and complementary practitioners move closer together, the ultimate benefit is the patient's. It would be a tragedy if the irresponsible, get-rich-quick merchants upset this delicately balanced apple cart.

It is time that the government took some action. After all, you have to be a registered farrier in order to shoe horses, so why can't there be a register of bona fide competent complementary practitioners? At the back of the book you will find a list of organisations from whom you can obtain registers of their practising members (page 287). Of course, the first person you should ask if you are seeking a complementary practitioner is your own GP, since he is much more likely to know who the local competent people are than the lady in the corner shop.

For those of you interested in pursuing the knowledge of complementary therapies further, you will find a reading list at the back of the book (page 285). You may be surprised at how many of these books are related to food and nutrition. You may also be surprised to see how frequently the question of healthy eating crops up during the text of this book. The reason for this is not hard to find.

How great is the British diet?

In spite of all the recent publicity given to the food that we eat, the food that we do not eat and the food that we should eat, the vast majority of the great British public do not live on a healthy balanced diet.

A recent report in England looked at the eating habits of more than 800 people in nearly 500 households and came up with some startling facts. In spite of the supposed interest in better eating, the report found that 93 per cent of all men and 98 per cent of women between the ages of 18 and 54 do not have enough folate in their diet. Folates are the body's source of essential folic acid, a vital substance for blood formation and protein metabolism.

Sixty per cent of women between the ages of 18 and 54 do not get enough iron. Over 90 per cent of all men and women do not get enough of vitamin B6. B6 or pyridoxine, known as the anti-depression vitamin, is extremely important, especially for women on the pill, smokers, regular alcohol drinkers, and for the treatment of premenstrual tension.

The diet of 73 per cent of all women contained less calcium than the recommended daily quantities and calcium is essential for the proper formation of bones, teeth, nails and hair. It is especially important for women after the menopause when they can lose calcium from their bones, and for pregnant and nursing mothers whose demand for calcium increases. The survey also found that 57 per cent of all women had a zinc intake below the levels recommended by the World Health Organisation. Zinc deficiency can lead to a wide range of health problems: lack of physical, mental and sexual development, poor appetite, slow healing of wounds and injuries, and – in men – impotence.

Finally the survey also found that the average amount of fibre in the diet of all the people surveyed was only 20 grams for men and 18 grams for women, whilst 30 grams per day is the minimum amount of fibre recommended.

How do you measure up in the vitamin stakes? Do you eat lots of take-aways? Do you feed your children on convenience foods and frozen TV dinners? Is your idea of fresh fruit a tangerine in the Christmas stocking? Does your diet contain lots of refined processed starchy foods, instant puddings, synthetic trifles, packet soups? Eating well is not difficult, not cranky, not expensive, if you follow these simple rules:

(1) One-third of your food should be raw fresh produce – fruit, salads, vegetables. Raw foods are a valuable source of fibre, vitamins and minerals.
(2) Use wholemeal bread, wholemeal pasta and brown rice for fibre and protein.
(3) Poultry and fish are healthy sources of protein, red meats should have the fat removed and preferably be grilled.

Dairy products and eggs are valuable additions to any diet but should be used with common sense. A little pure butter is far better than masses of chemical margarine which has the same number of calories.

Avoid expensive processed foods and use home-made soups, beans of all sorts and vegetable casseroles as an occasional alternative to meat. Cut down on all meat products – sausages, pies, salamis, pâtés – all of which contain huge amounts of hidden fats.

You do not need to be a food freak, a crank or even a vegetarian to be healthy, although a good vegetarian diet has been shown to be better for overall health than a meat-eating diet. All you need is a little thought and a lot of common sense.

You will find lots more dietary information later on in the book and sometimes you may think that the advice seems to be rather extreme. This is always for a very specific reason. It is occasionally a therapeutic necessity to follow a vegetarian diet or to fast or to cut certain substances totally out of your daily food intake, like dairy products, foods containing wheat, or those which are likely to contain yeast. Apart from these specific instances, the overall nutritional message in this book is one of balance. There is a sensible and healthy half-way house between the Big Mac and Coca-Cola addict and the health food freak who lives on nothing but brown rice and a grated carrot.

In my own practice I have often found it easier to deal with the hamburger and cola addict, since it is not hard to point out the error of their ways to somebody whose diet is basically one of foods of predominantly low nutrient density, whereas the health food freaks consider themselves to be on some form of holy quest. These people frequently follow diets which do not provide an adequate daily intake of the essential nutrients and serious problems can occur when they try to bring up children on these same extreme nutritional programmes.

There is a very definite swing away from meat eating in this country. The Vegetarian Society calculates that there are now more than one million real vegetarians and another million who eat fish and poultry but avoid red meats. This latter group has been termed 'demi-veg' and a growing number of cookery books are appearing aimed at this new group of healthier eaters.

There is considerable evidence to show that following a good vegetarian diet is healthier than being a meat eater. When I recently visited Harvard University Medical School one of the professors who runs the cholesterol research laboratory there told me that in his surveys there was no doubt at all that the vegetarians they studied at Harvard had a lower incidence of coronary heart disease, a lower incidence of high blood pressure and a much lower level of blood cholesterol compared with a sample of meat eaters.

The moral vegetarian, however, is rather more at risk than the health vegetarian. In this country we have many people who decide to become vegetarians for purely moral reasons. This includes large numbers of young teenage girls and, whilst the genuine motives for their decision cannot be questioned, I am sometimes rather alarmed by their lack of nutritional knowledge. I receive many letters from mothers who are extremely concerned about their daughters' overall level of nutrition when they decide to stop eating meat and, judging by some of the diet sheets which some of these mothers send me, the concern is not at all misplaced.

If you or someone in your family decides to become a vegetarian, do make sure that you acquire sufficient knowledge to do it healthily. The Vegetarian Society runs cookery courses, lectures, and provides some extremely useful literature, and of course there are many excellent vegetarian cookery books ranging from Chinese vegetarian cookery right the way through to Jewish vegetarian cookery, and you will find a large selection in your local health food store and bookshop.

If you're going to be a vegetarian it's vital that you learn to do it properly. There are lots of old wives' tales about the evils that will follow if you don't eat plenty of meat. None of them are true, even though they are often trotted out by doctors, mothers-in-law and grannies. Just last year the Minister of Agriculture issued a statement that 'it is dangerous for women to be vegetarians'. One can only assume that the meat-producing agricultural lobby had a hand in putting their foot in his mouth! You will not be weak or stupid if you stop eating meat, nor will you become impotent if you are a man, or infertile if you're a woman. Billions of people throughout the world are healthy, strong, virile, fertile, intelligent and active vegetarians.

There is no need to consume vast quantities of synthetic meat substitutes like TVP, Quorn, Vegeburgers, Vegebangers or other commercially produced vegetarian foods. There's nothing wrong with them and some are quite palatable, but they are expensive and they are not necessary. What you need from any healthy diet is energy, which is obtained from a mixture of foods providing protein, fats, carbohydrates, vitamins and minerals. The wider the variety of foods that you eat, the less likely you are to be deficient in any of the essential nutrients. Just because you remove meat, fish and poultry from your daily meals there is no reason to worry about your health; in fact it is likely to be a great deal better without the intake of saturated animal fats. Vitamins D and B12 are the only nutrients which may cause a problem but this is easily overcome (see under Vitamins).

Children and teenagers need a high energy diet and this can sometimes be a problem if they are vegetarians. Make sure that they have plenty of high energy foods and not too much of the very bulky foods which may fill them up but leave them short of calories. Dairy products, nuts, seeds, fats and oils provide more calories and less bulk. For this reason bringing up children on a totally vegan diet, that is without eggs or any dairy products, can be difficult and I certainly do not recommend it. In order to get 500 calories you need to eat five slices of bread, 140 grams of rice, 185 grams of dried beans, but only 90 grams of nuts, 70 grams of butter, 55 grams of oil or 120 grams of cheddar cheese.

Protein has always been the vexed question of vegetarianism. Animal sources of protein including dairy products and soya are the most efficiently used by the body. Other forms of protein from cereals, pulses and nuts are not dealt with quite so well. During the process of digestion proteins are broken down into their constituent amino acids which are what the body absorbs. Apart from soya protein, none of the other plant sources contain all the essential amino acids and for this reason it has been suggested that vegetarians don't get enough protein. As long as your diet contains a mixture of different vegetable protein sources, it will provide you with all the protein you need. If you include some dairy products and soya, either as beans, flour or tofu, you will have nothing to worry about.

The meat eaters amongst you will be surprised to learn that mixing cereals and pulses, for example baked beans on wholemeal toast or kidney beans and rice, provides the same quality of protein as a fillet steak. What's more, for protein quality the potato scores 70 out of 100, oatmeal scores 65 and meat scores only 80. The best score goes to the humble egg which, together with mother's milk, score the maximum 100.

Provided your diet contains fruit, vegetables, whole cereals and grains and nuts, you will get adequate amounts of vitamins A, B complex, C and E. Vitamin D is not available from vegetable sources, but is added to margarine and is manufactured by the body when the skin is exposed to sunlight. Elderly vegetarians, who may not go out much during cold weather, and vegetarian children, should both be given a vitamin D supplement in winter. The only other problem may arise with vitamin B12. Eggs are a good source but note that free range eggs contain considerably more, 2.9 micrograms per 100 grams, than battery eggs which only supply 1.7 micrograms per 100 grams. Yeast extracts also contain small amounts of this vitamin but even vegetarians who eat eggs and dairy products should take a B12 supplement regularly, and I believe it's essential for vegans.

Minerals are another essential component of the diet. Calcium, essential for the proper formation of bones, is not likely to be a problem for vegetarians who include dairy products. There are quite good vegetable sources of calcium especially molasses, sesame seeds, beans, broccoli and most nuts. Although spinach contains a lot of calcium, it also contains oxalates which combine with calcium to form an insoluble salt which the body can't use. A similar problem occurs with the chemical phytic acid which is found in wheat and also combines with calcium. The effect of yeast and cooking in breadmaking destroys the phytic acid, but sprinkling spoonsful of bran on top of your cornflakes is not a good idea as the bran has a high concentration of phytic acid. Calcium is particularly important for young women as the sound development of strong bones in the 20s and 30s can be a great advantage after the menopause when the possibility of osteoporosis looms.

Most doctors seem to worry about their vegetarian patients becoming anaemic as everyone associates iron with meat and liver. There is plenty of iron in wholemeal bread, good cereals and dark green leafy vegetables which the careful vegetarian will be eating in abundance. Since the absorption of iron is greatly improved in the presence of vitamin C, and again, because the good vegetarian will also be consuming much more fresh fruit than the average meat eater, anaemia is a rare problem in all but the worst vegetarians.

For many years vegetarian food in the UK has been dismal compared to that in the rest of the world. We have a surplus of what I have dubbed 'pudding vegetarians'. They become vegetarian for moral reasons and have little interest in nutrition, unlike most European vegetarians who tend to be more concerned with the health benefits. We have recently heard much more about the Mediterranean diet which includes wonderful dishes that happen not to contain meat or fish: tasty pasta prepared with vegetables like artichokes and spinach; imaginative salads combining the freshest of leaves with fragrant herbs like mint, basil and coriander; dishes made with peppers, aubergines and olives; and the delights of olive oil, garlic and coarse country breads.

Food must look, smell and taste wonderful if we are going to enjoy eating it. A diet of endless stodgy nut roasts, cheesy bakes and leaden wholemeal pasta will not tempt many palates. Happily, some of the best chefs in England now offer delicious vegetarian dishes on their menus, better than in most vegetarian restaurants. Many a carnivore has been tempted by meat-free delights created by Anton Mosimann, Raymond Blanc, Antony Worrall Thompson and Prue Leith. For all their good intentions, maybe the moral vegetarians could convince greater numbers of people to eat less meat if they concentrated more on the tempting tastes and the health benefits than on the horrors of meat production.

Foods that could save your life

More than 2000 years ago, Hippocrates said, 'Let your food be your medicine, and your medicine be your food.' Now, as we reach the last decade of the 20th century, scientists are beginning to understand that the food we eat each day can make the difference between life and death.

No, I am not talking about the starving millions in the third world, but those of us right here in Great Britain.

The truth is that though an apple a day might keep the doctor away, eating more fresh fruit, salad and vegetables will keep you out of the hospital. Evidence collected from worldwide studies shows us that those people whose diets are rich in these simple, inexpensive foods are less likely to suffer from heart disease and cancer.

Compared with the rest of Europe, the inhabitants of this 'Green and pleasant land' come top of the league table for heart disease and some types of cancer. At the same time, we are at the very bottom of the tables for the consumption of fresh fruit and vegetables. Just to give you some idea of the scale of the problem, a middle-aged man in Scotland is five times more likely to die from heart disease than his equal living in the south of France!

How is it that something as simple as eating more fruit and vegetables is now seen as a way of protecting ourselves from the ravages of cancer and heart disease? For many years, practitioners of alternative medicine have argued that there is a great difference between getting enough vitamins to prevent deficiency diseases, like scurvy or rickets – these amounts are known as the Recommended Dietary Allowances, or RDAs – and the quantity we need for optimum health.

At last the scientists have realised that we do need more of these essential micronutrients in order to combat the destructive 'free radicals' which are now known to play a major part in many diseases. Vitamins C, E and beta-carotene exert a powerful protective effect, as they are 'antioxidants' and can neutralise the dangerous 'free radicals'.

Where do we find the richest sources of these vital substances? In fruit and vegetables. Most of us don't eat enough of them to supply the minimum needs, let alone the quantities that give us the extra protection, which studies from all over the world clearly show to be the first step along the road to better health.

Free radicals and antioxidants

Free radicals are the villains of the piece. They are produced by our bodies as the by-product of some of the normal chemical processes which happen all the time. These free radicals are biologically active, and very destructive substances, so it is vital that they are removed as quickly as possible. If not, they combine with oxygen and cause severe damage to body cells – the same process which makes butter turn rancid when left out of the fridge.

Antioxidants are the heroes. They act as scavengers, cleaning the system of the free radicals, and protecting the body from their destructive power.

Vitamin C, vitamin E and beta-carotene are three of the most important antioxidants. They help to protect the body against heart disease and some types of cancer. You can get all you need of these vital nutrients by eating enough of the right foods.

Heart disease

Nearly one-third of all deaths in the UK are the result of heart disease. Someone, more often male, will die every three minutes of the day and night, and most of these deaths are premature and preventable.

Total deaths from heart disease is like a full Jumbo jet crashing at Heathrow Airport, each day of the week, and two on Sundays, throughout the year!

There are many causes of heart disease, but the most common is the result of a reduction in the supply of blood to the heart muscle itself. This is due to the narrowing of the arteries to the heart because they become hardened and the walls get thicker – arteriosclerosis – or by the deposit of fat on the inside of the artery walls – atherosclerosis.

Both of these conditions are the result of a combination of factors over a long period of time. Family history of heart disease, smoking, too much alcohol, too much animal fat, too little fibre, too much salt, too little exercise and too much stress. The end result is that free radicals attack one of the protective substances in the blood, LDL (low-density lipoprotein), and this is the start of the problem. LDL is itself protected from damage by the presence of vitamin E.

Increasing the amount of antioxidants in the blood helps to prevent heart disease. Vitamin E would appear to be the most important of them in order to reduce the risk of damaging arteries carrying blood to the heart muscle.

Cancer

Most of the cells that make up all our body tissues are able to divide and multiply. This is a normal, everyday happening, but the way in which cells do this is strictly controlled by special genes. When these genes become damaged, they may lose their ability to stop the division of cells and this is when problems can start.

There are many causes of cancer, not one single factor. But in the end, it is the uncontrolled multiplication of a group of cells that is 'cancer'. Free radicals can attack and injure the genes which regulate cell division. So, it is important to give the body as much protection as possible, and the antioxidant properties of vitamin C and beta-carotene appear to be vital in this respect.

Beta-carotene

Studies in Europe, Japan and the USA strongly suggest that high levels of beta-carotene consumption, in the form of fruit and vegetables, are linked with a reduced risk of lung cancer and cancers of the digestive system.

Vitamin C

Throughout the world investigations show that eating plenty of the vitamin C rich foods will give added protection against cancers of the mouth, throat, cervix and breast.

41

Vitamin E

The World Health Organisation has examined sixteen population groups around Europe. They found that the lower the amount of vitamin E in the blood of the volunteers, the greater their risk of dying from heart disease.

The Fresh Fruit and Vegetable Information Bureau asked Dr Kevin Cheeseman, from Brunel University, to make a study of all the scientific literature on the role of antioxidants as a protection against disease. His conclusion is: 'Strong and convincing evidence from studies carried out around the world show that a diet rich in fruit and vegetables is associated with a low incidence of heart disease and certain cancers. The active ingredients responsible for these beneficial effects are most probably beta-carotene and vitamins C and E, acting as natural antioxidants and helping to prevent the slow accumulation of damage that is characteristic of chronic diseases.'

The American Department of Health recommends that everyone should eat a total of five portions of fresh fruit and vegetables, each day. Very few of us here in the UK get anywhere near that amount, in spite of the evidence that the whole nation would be healthier if we did.

You can reduce the risks of heart disease and some types of cancer, for yourself and your family, by the simple, cheap and enjoyable act of making sure you all eat much more fresh fruit and vegetables.

There are two positive advantages to eating more of this nature's bounty. As well as increasing your consumption of all the things which actively promote good health, you will have less room to fill up with all those sweet and fatty foods: the baddies which sow the seeds of future problems.

Use the following chart to make sure that you are eating enough of the right foods to get your share of the antioxidants. To obtain your daily requirement of vitamin C, vitamin E and beta-carotene, simply tot up the percentages of a good selection of the foods listed. If you want your health to be 100 per cent, aim for the magic total of 100 per cent for each of these essential nutrients.

BETA-CAROTENE

100 g of	percentage of daily requirement
fresh apricots	19
cantaloupe melon	15
carrots – new	75
carrots – old	150
lettuce – 50 g	6

mango	15
parsley – 50 g	44
peach	5
spinach	75
sprouts	50
tomato	7

VITAMIN C

100 g of	**percentage of daily requirement**
blackcurrants	400
cauliflower	120
gooseberries	80
kiwi	196
lemon	160
lettuce – 50 g	15
melon	30
orange	76
green pepper	200
potatoes	36
radish – 50 g	25
sprouts	80
strawberries	120
tomato	40
turnip	34
watercress – 50 g	60

VITAMIN E

100 g of	**percentage of daily requirement**
apple	2
asparagus	25
avocado – half	30
banana	2
blackcurrants	10
broccoli	11
carrots	5
damsons	6
hazel nuts	85
parsley – 50 g	9
spinach	20
sunflower seed oil – 5 g	30
sweet potato	50
tomato	12
watercress – 50 g	5

Additives – yellow for danger

The question of food additives is another subject which you will find cropping up repeatedly throughout the book. For many years complementary practitioners, and especially naturopaths like myself, have been extremely concerned about the growing use of artificial additives which are being consumed in ever growing quantities. Yet again it is the public who have forced both the medical profession and the food manufacturers to take greater note of the growing concern about these dubious chemicals. In his book *E for Additives*, Maurice Hanssen gives a complete list of all the additives legally used in the food industry in this country and, in spite of the fact that this book topped the best seller lists for several weeks, many, many people throughout the United Kingdom are still unaware, not only of the dangers of these chemicals, but even of their presence in the everyday foods which we eat. Does this sound familiar?

You've just about cleared up the dirty dishes after lunch, you have finished the ironing and you sit down for a quiet cup of tea before the kids come charging home from school. You pick up the knife, you cut a large thick slice of cake and nibble contentedly:

E440 (A)	Liquid pectin, a gelling agent and emulsifier. Can cause stomach distention and flatulence.
Modified starch	A thickener.
E465	Ethylmethylcellulose – a stabiliser and emulsifier.
E471	Mono-diglycerides – emulsifier and stabiliser.
E330	Citric acid – prevents discolouration. Large quantities can damage tooth enamel.
E331	Sodium citrate – anti-oxidant.
E102	Tartrazine – yellow colour. Has serious effects on food-sensitive children, causes sleeplessness, hyperactivity, skin rashes, blurred vision and is particularly irritant to asthmatics or aspirin-sensitive people. Can trigger asthma attacks.
E110	Sunset yellow – yellow colouring. Irritant to hyperactive children, can produce allergies in adults, especially skin rashes and stomach problems in those sensitive to aspirin.
E123	Amaranth – red colour, causes skin rashes in aspirin-sensitive people and aggravates hyperactivity in children.
E124	Ponceau 4R – red colouring. Can affect asthmatics and hyperactive children.
Flavouring	Many synthetic flavours can cause adverse reactions.

E202   Potassium sorbate – preservative.
E282   Calcium propionate – preservative.

You have just eaten a delicious slice of swiss roll and I am sure that you didn't read the label before you bought it and now that you know what is in it I hope that you will throw it away before the children come home.

Most food additives provide nothing of nutritional value and are only there for the convenience of the manufacturers and the retailers, as by using them they can produce foods with a longer shelf life and manufacture products using cheaper ingredients or smaller quantities of the more expensive ones.

In 1970 I met an American allergist, Dr Ben Finegold, the first to suggest a link between abnormal behaviour in children and food additives, and I invited him to lecture here in England. It was twelve years before the medical profession in this country took any real notice of the dangers of additives, whilst practitioners of alternative medicine had been consistently warning about the problems. It is certain that many asthmatic and allergic children suffer severe consequences as a result of eating foods containing additives. It is also certain that many non-allergic people suffer some adverse reactions to the chemicals in the food they eat every day. In spite of what the proponents of food additives say, the majority of these chemicals are not tested or even under the control of government departments, and the best advice is to try and avoid all of them wherever possible. This is even more important if anybody in your family is known to suffer from allergies.

Some retailers are behaving far more responsibly than the manufacturers by trying to reduce the level of additives in the foods which they sell. Tesco's, for instance, have started a nutritional labelling scheme in their stores and are introducing lines containing fewer chemicals. They are particularly aiming to exclude tartrazine from all foods sold in their stores as soon as possible, as well as giving the shopper more information about sugar, salt, fat and fibre contents for food.

It is only when more of you stop buying the junk foods that the manufacturers will be forced into providing an alternative.

E for effort not additives

(1) Make the effort to be a label reader. Not all E brands are bad, some are natural products, learn to tell the difference.
(2) Avoid the worst offenders – squash, fizzy drinks, brightly coloured sweets, lollipops, ice lollies.
(3) Avoid highly processed packaged foods like instant trifles,

instant desserts, whips and puddings. These are some of the worst offenders and aimed directly at the children's mind.

(4) Nag your local shopkeepers to carry a wider range of foods that are free from additives.

(5) Do not spend more money – whilst health food shops provide an excellent source of many pure foods, more and more supermarkets are selling products without additives at lower prices.

(6) If you think your child suffers from adverse reactions to additives, keep these out of the diet and don't be put off by anyone. You can get help and advice from The Hyperactive Children's Support Group, 59 Meadowside, Angmering, West Sussex.

You will find a more complete list of the most important additives later on in the book (page 274) and specific reference to them in the appropriate sections relating to individual symptoms.

Herbs for health and beauty

Since time began, man has turned to the world of plants to provide relief from his aches and pains, and to soothe away the ravages of wind and weather on his skin. There is no inhabited area of our globe that has not yielded some plants from which medicines can be made.

Even in one grave of Neanderthal man, unearthed in Iraq after 60,000 years, pollen grains from eight different flowers were found scattered around the bones. Seven of these are still in common use today as medicines.

How did our ancestors know which plants to use? Certainly there must have been disasters, herbal products which, at best, did not work, and at worst, produced a fatal outcome. But there must also have been some instinctive understanding, similar to that which animals seem to possess. You only need to watch your cat or dog to see how they sniff out a particular plant to chew, when they are ill. How else would it be possible that tribes of natives as far apart as Fiji, Samoa, India, Trinidad and Vietnam, could all use the same remedy – hibiscus tea – for menstrual problems and for the control of fertility? What is even more surprising is that it probably worked! The particular hibiscus they all used has marked anti-oestrogen properties.

The use of medicinal herbs spread throughout the world. Some 3000 years before Christ, the Chinese had written down their prescriptions; 1000 years later, the Babylonians carved their herbal knowledge on to tablets of stone. From the Ganges to the Nile, information and materials were exchanged and traded.

Many new medicines were brought to England by the Roman armies, who never travelled without a supply of plants and seeds. The first thing that their physicians did when a new garrison was established was to plant a herb garden, including mustard and garlic, later to become staples of the British herbalists.

The Welsh Druids, monks and the traditions of folk-lore all added to our body of information, and herbal medicine flourished up to the early 20th century. But it was the great Prussian biochemist, Paul Ehrlich, who sounded the death knell with his 'Magic Bullets' concept of 'a pill for every ill'. And from here on, the pharmaceutical industry was on the path to domination of the entire drug scene.

There can be no denying that many drugs have made untold contributions to the welfare and survival of sick people: antibiotics, painkillers, anti-inflammatories and all the other preparations which everyone would agree are indispensable. But sadly, this has caused the entire field of herbal medicine to be rejected, and condemned as folk-lore and mumbo jumbo. This, in spite of the fact that many of the major 'new' drugs were derived from plant material. Even now, some 25 per cent of prescriptions contain at least one important ingredient from the herbal world. Digoxin, quinine, morphine, atropine, codeine, ephedrine and vincristine are just some of these in everyday use.

Quack or cure?

With a few notable exceptions, like belladonna and the other deadly poisons, herbal medicines are safe and effective. Yet the majority of doctors dismiss these gifts from nature as 'quack' cures. They regard all plant preparations as little more than old wives' tales, and continue to prescribe larger and larger quantities of drugs which often have side effects. There are many situations when the gentler action of herbs and the lack of unwanted counter effects would be more appropriate. People have become uneasy about the over-use of powerful drugs and are themselves turning to the plant world for the treatment of their minor ailments.

At the same time, there is a revolution going on in the scientific investigation of these preparations. Research is now able to prove just how often the old wives were right, and in many cases, bear out the wisdom of the ancient herbalists.

Garlic, one of the most used of medicinal plants, is now firmly established as a potent protector against heart disease. Large-scale clinical trials have shown that Kwai garlic tablets sharply reduced the death rate in a study of 400 patients who had already suffered one heart attack. It lowered cholesterol levels, reduced blood pressure, improved circulation and reduced the tendency to form blood clots. (For more detailed information see end of this chapter.)

Evening primrose oil, which so many women have found relieves their PMS, has been the subject of many experiments, using Efamol, which demonstrate that it helps in a wide range of other conditions. Multiple sclerosis, diabetes, heart and circulatory disease, obesity, Raynaud's syndrome, rheumatoid disease, and particularly eczema (for which it may now be prescribed on the NHS) can all benefit from this humble plant.

Without doubt, the pioneer and leading figure in the scientific testing of herbal medicines is the remarkable Swiss, Fred Pestalozzi. Nearly forty years ago he was an engineer working in his home town of Zurich. His own experience of an incurable illness which was 'cured' by a herbal medicine led him to give up his work in the family firm, and, starting from scratch in 1961, he built the company which produces Bio-Strath Elixir.

From the outset, he was determined that his product would be a meeting of two worlds – the ancient world of traditional herbal wisdom and the modern world of scientific research. All the plants are tested to ensure that they contain the vital active substances, and the end product, made without heat or artificial ingredients, is tested again to confirm that they are still there.

Pestalozzi was intent on proving beyond doubt that Bio-Strath was both safe and effective. He initiated a research programme on a scale never seen before in the herbal world. Scientists from universities and independent laboratories in England, Switzerland and Germany were persuaded to work on the experiments. At first they were all sceptical, but soon became enthusiastic as the results of their studies emerged.

This simple combination of medicinal herbs, a special strain of yeast, orange juice and honey, has been shown to have far-reaching benefits. It can increase performance, speed convalescence, protect against the side effects of radiotherapy, increase the number of white cells in the blood, and so improve the body's immune defences against everyday infections. The latest trials have shown that Bio-Strath has a protective effect in the treatment of 'pre' Alzheimer's disease. All these without any unwanted side effects. Results of this work have been published in the scientific journals, and have set a benchmark for the entire herbal industry.

Bio-Strath also led the way in the field of specific medicines. It was the first company to be granted licences for herbal preparations. A vast research programme produced the evidence to satisfy the Department of Health that their six products for the treatment of individual problems were safe and effective. The products were artichoke formula for indigestion after fatty foods; liquorice formula for aiding the digestion; thyme formula for coughs;

chamomile formula for mouth and throat problems; valerian formula for nervousness and stress; and willow formula for back ache, lumbago, fibrositis and muscle pain. And in 1992 a licence was granted for the tonic preparation, Bio-Strath Elixir.

Fred Pestalozzi has a simple philosophy: 'Without scientific proof there will be no future survival for herbal medicines.'

Simple herbal remedies for everyday ailments

A trip to any health food store, or your nearest pharmacy, will lead you to shelves of herbal medicines. If you need more expert help, then you can consult a medical herbalist – look for the letters MNIMH after the name to be sure that the practitioner you choose has been trained and is qualified. Even your local supermarket will have a wide selection of herbal teas and fresh herbs. You may think that these are just a way of avoiding caffeine, or for use in cooking, but they can often have powerful medicinal actions.

The folk-lore of herbs has always been a part of 'kitchen medicine', so here is my list of the top remedies that you can make at home, and use to treat a range of minor family ailments. All of the following recipes are safe and effective. As with all forms of self-medication, if the symptoms persist, or worsen, seek advice from your own GP.

Acne Drink three cups of nettle tea each day. Make each cup fresh from a heaped teaspoon of chopped nettle leaves, on to which pour a cupful of boiling water. Cover and leave to stand for two minutes, strain and sip slowly.

Catarrh Eat lots of garlic, or take two Kwai garlic tablets, three times daily. Make an infusion of hyssop, using the leaves, stem and flowers. Sweeten with honey and drink a cup three times daily.

Colds At the first sign of a cold, add a heaped teaspoon of dried English mustard to half a bucket of hot water. Sit with feet in the bucket for at least ten minutes, just before bedtime. To ease the symptoms, make an infusion of elder flowers, add a pinch of cayenne pepper, a pinch of cinnamon and a little freshly grated ginger root. Drink this fiery mixture just before you go to bed, and prepare for a hot, sweaty night. You will feel better by morning.

Corns and fungal infections Corns and fungal infections of the toe and finger nails all respond to the power of the nettle. Use as foot or hand baths and prepare with ten whole stems with leaves on, soaked in 4 pints of cold water for an hour, then warmed up gently till they are comfortably hot. Soak the hands or feet for at least half an hour daily.

A tincture of nettle roots can be painted on to corns or infected nails. Make it by filling a half-size wine bottle with finely chopped roots, add alcohol – gin or vodka are fine – to the top, and cork tightly. Leave for three weeks, then use as required.

Coughs One of the best cough medicines is elecampane root. Simmer half an ounce in one pint of water for twenty minutes. Strain, and while still hot, add a tablespoon of clear honey and the juice of two lemons. Stir well and take a warm wineglassful, three times a day. Another old-wives' favourite is garlic and honey. Thinly slice eight to ten peeled cloves of garlic and add them to a pound jar of clear honey. Leave for at least twenty-four hours, then take a teaspoon or two each hour. It really tastes better than it sounds!

Cystitis If you suspect a urinary infection, see your doctor. But, as millions of women know, antibiotics do not always help this condition. Here's a remedy which will allay much of the discomfort. Pour a cupful of boiling water on to a teaspoon of powdered marshmallow root. Stir, and leave for twenty minutes. Add one teaspoon of honey, and take the resulting paste three times a day, before meals.

Digestive problems To relieve flatulence or nausea, chew a few fresh basil leaves, or a little nutmeg, simmered in half a cup of milk with a teaspoon of honey. For stomach cramp, take a cup of hot peppermint tea. For severe indigestion, or for inflammation after a gastric upset, mix a teaspoon of slippery elm powder into a paste, using a little cold water. Add a pinch of cinnamon and some honey, together with a cup of boiling water. Take two or three cups daily. For acid stomach, make some meadowsweet tea, and sip slowly after meals.

Healing cream For dry, sore, chapped or otherwise damaged skin, make an infusion of comfrey and marigold leaves, one teaspoon of each chopped, covered with a cup of boiling water, and left to stand for ten minutes. Strain, and add to it enough aqueous cream (from any chemist) to make a rich smooth cream. Add a few drops of almond oil and the content of four vitamin E capsules. Keep in a tightly closed jar, in the fridge.

Insomnia Chamomile, catnip or hop teas are simple and effective. Use a hop-filled pillow, or add some Kneipp hop oil to your bedtime bath. Make a strong infusion of any of these teas, and add that to your bath. Surprisingly, orange blossom is one of the best of all soporifics: apart from its popularity in bridal bouquets, it makes a delicious tea. Take fifty drops of Bio-Strath valerian formula.

Migraine The herbal star in the treatment of this wretched illness is, without doubt, feverfew. You can grow it in the garden, or in a windowbox, and two leaves a day is usually enough. Do take it in a sandwich, as it can cause mouth ulcers in some people. Feverfew tablets are available from health stores. Lime flower or peppermint tea are good too, and it helps to add a sprig of dried lavender. Eucalyptus, rosemary or lavender oil, massaged into the forehead and temples, will help with the pain.

Sore throats Gargle with a cup of red sage tea, adding a teaspoon of cider vinegar. Repeat four or five times daily, and swallow one or two mouthfuls each time. Thyme is a good alternative if you don't have any sage.

Baby colic Commercial gripe waters are available, but it is best to make your own – it's also a lot cheaper. Use dill, fennel or caraway seeds. Crush a level teaspoon of seeds between two spoons or with a rolling pin, soak in a cup of boiling water for half an hour, strain and use one teaspoonful as a relieving dose.

Nappy rash Calendula (marigold) ointment is both soothing and healing. You may also use an infusion of elder flowers. Add a teaspoon of dried flowers, or two of fresh, to a pint of boiling water. Cover and leave for twenty minutes, then when cool, dip a sterile gauze into the tea, wring out and apply to the sore areas.

General information

To make teas (infusions) use one teaspoon of the dried herb, or two if using fresh, place in a small teapot, a special 'infuser' or a mug. Add a cupful of boiling water, cover to preserve the volatile oils and leave for ten minutes. Strain – I use one of the paper coffee filters – add a little honey if you wish, and drink warm, three times a day before meals.

Many of the herbs are available both fresh and dried from the herb section of your local supermarket, greengrocer or corner shop. The medicinal ones may be found at the chemist or health store, but you can get them by post from some of the herbal suppliers like Culpeper Ltd., Hadstock Road, Linton, Cambridge, or Neal's Yard Apothecary, 2 Neal's Yard, Covent Garden, London WC2.

More information on herbs from The Herb Society, 77 Great Peter Street, London SW1.

For details of qualified herbalists, contact the National Institute of Medical Herbalists, PO Box 3, Winchester SO22 6RR.

Herbs for skin and hair care

Cleopatra bathed in asses' milk in order to make her skin more beautiful. It's certain that she also used a whole range of natural plant extracts both as make-up and to look after her skin and hair. After all, she lived in the dry, dusty and sun-drenched atmosphere of Egypt, and you know what havoc such conditions can wreak on the complexion. What's more, she didn't have Boots or the Body Shop just around the corner.

Here is a complete guide to taking care of your skin and hair. All the ingredients that you need to make your own preparations can be found in your chemist, health store, supermarket, green-grocer or from the herbal suppliers listed (page 51). They are simple to make, cheap, free from artificial additives which may be irritant, and are environment friendly. You will have the added pleasure of knowing that no animals have suffered in the preparation of your cosmetics.

Cleanliness is next to Godliness, so they say, and it is surely true that no skin care regime will be a success unless you start with a clean skin.

Start your cleansing programme with a good old-fashioned steam bath. You don't need a fancy electric facial steamer – just a bowl, a towel and a kettle of boiling water. Add a few herbs to the water and you have the ideal combination.

Use a heaped teaspoon of the relevant herb, place in a large mixing bowl, pour on a kettle full of boiling water, cover your head and the bowl with a large towel, and sit in the steam for ten minutes. **Do not use this method if you have thread veins or very delicate skin!** For general cleansing use elderflowers; for cleansing and soothing, a mixture of chamomile and lavender; for city grime limeflowers are best; rosemary stimulates the circulation; peppermint tightens the skin; fennel will help to heal any scars or blemishes.

After this process, make sure that you close up the pores by rubbing the skin with a chunk of peeled cucumber, or dabbing with cold chamomile tea.

One of the oldest known cleansers is made according to this recipe: to eight fluid ounces of boiled, cooled water add twenty drops of simple tincture of benzoin, and four drops each of tincture of myrrh and glycerine. Shake well before use, and store in a stoppered bottle in the fridge.

For greasy skin, use a carton of natural yoghurt with half a teaspoon of coarse sea salt stirred into it.

A real boon for those with sensitive skin is bran or oatmeal. Make a small bag from a strip of muslin, fill it with one of these, soak in warm water and use to wash the face. After four or five washes, empty and replace with fresh contents.

They both contain vitamin E and vegetable mucilage to encourage the skin.

Facials   Even the oldest of herbal books give some recipes for facial masks – wanting to look your best is not a modern trait. Here's one which doubles as healing and nourishing. Place a carton of natural yoghurt into a bowl, add one capsule each of vitamins A and E (pierce them with a pin and squeeze out the contents), one teaspoon of sesame seed oil, two dessertspoons of avocado and wheatgerm oil, one tablespoon of almond oil and two drops of lavender oil. Mix thoroughly and apply to the face. Leave on for half to one hour. Wash off gently with warm water.

Use a parsley facial to give your skin that healthy glow. Boil a handful of fresh parsley in half a pint of water for ten minutes. Strain, then mix the cooled water with a tablespoon of honey and a stiffly beaten egg white. Apply and leave on the face for twenty minutes. Wash off with warm water.

Spots   Can be a nightmare, so try this simple cream. You'll need one large apple, peeled and cored, two tablespoons each of chopped fennel bulb and celery, four egg whites, 2 pints of rose water, 1 ounce of bran, one teaspoon of anhydrous lanolin. Simmer all except the lanolin and egg whites until very soft. Add beaten whites and lanolin, then push through a sieve. Beat together till the mixture is smooth. Store in the fridge until required.

Another good spot treatment is vinegar. Don't worry, you are not going to smell like a chip, not if you use this recipe. To 1 pint of cider vinegar add 5 tablespoons of fresh lavender, rosemary or rose petals. Leave for three weeks, then add 2 pints of boiled, cooled water. Use this as a daily skin wash which is astringent and curative.

Hand care   When doing all those jobs around the house, wear gloves. It may seem obvious, but most women don't seem to bother, other than for washing up or cleaning the loo! Polishes, dust, dirt and grime will soon become ingrained into the skin and around the nails. It is much easier to keep them out than to get them off. Herb teas used for soaking a compress are great for restoring the chapped skin of work-worn hands. Use marigold petals, comfrey or chamomile.

To soften the cuticles, mix half a glass of fresh pineapple juice with one beaten egg yolk and a teaspoon of cider vinegar. Soak the finger tips in the mixture for half an hour.

It is worth making up a stock of your own herbal waters, as they can form the base for many other recipes. Prepare rose or orange water simply by adding half an ounce of pure plant essence to around 3 pints of distilled water. Keep in a tightly closed bottle for at least two weeks for the full aroma to penetrate.

Make a good hand and foot lotion by adding four tablespoons of glycerine to half a cup of orange or rose water. Keep in a bottle, and shake vigorously before use.

To make a really special lavender water, grind a tablespoon of dried lavender together with a tablespoon of cinnamon, in a pestle and mortar. Place in a stoppered bottle, with half a pint of ethyl alcohol or vodka, and leave to steep for three weeks. Strain through a coffee filter before use.

Hair herbs   You can make your own herbal shampoo with little trouble. As long as you start with a good quality product, it is simple. Use coconut, avocado or any other vegetable-based, low-detergent shampoo. If you have fair hair, you should add a strong infusion – two teaspoons of dried herb to a cup of boiling water – of chamomile or nettles. For dark hair use sage or rosemary.

A sheen-giving conditioner is made by boiling two tablespoons of fresh rosemary in a pint of water for ten minutes. Strain, then add 2 ounces of sweet almond oil and twenty drops of lavender oil. For the final rinse, add two tablespoons of cider vinegar and one of rose water to 2 pints of hot water. Work thoroughly through the hair.

A hair tonic can be prepared from 8 ounces of vodka, 2 ounces of nettles, 1 ounce of rosemary, 1 ounce of marigold petals, three drops of lavender oil and 4 ounces of distilled water. Add all the herbs to the vodka and leave for three weeks. Then add the lavender oil and water. Massage into the hair and scalp three times a week.

Dandruff will respond to a daily massage with nettle tonic. Make with four tablespoons of nettle leaves steeped in boiling water, and left to soak for four hours. Strain and add half a cup of lavender cider vinegar.

For men   Here are a couple of good skin tonics suitable for use as after-shave lotions. Wet shaving can leave the skin dry due to the soap, so use this soothing mixture. Add a teaspoon of dried, or two of fresh, sage and rosemary to 8 fluid ounces of cider vinegar. Keep in a screw-top bottle for two weeks. Strain off the herbs, return to the bottle and add 8 ounces of witch hazel.

A mildly perfumed lotion can be prepared from 2 ounces of fresh leaves from any variety of scented geranium. Wash and chop the leaves and add them to a pint of cider vinegar. Leave for two weeks in a screw-top bottle, filter off the leaves, add half a pint of distilled water.

Cooking with herbs

Perhaps there *was* a time when a bayleaf accidentally dropped into a caveman's cooking pot and set new standards in brontosaurus stew. Nobody knows exactly when – or why – our ancestors started to add leaves, roots and berries to their recipes, but there can't be a food lover throughout the world who isn't grateful that they did.

Herbs can transform the humblest stew into a casserole of elegance, give piquancy to the poorest cut of meat or fish, turn vegetables into a dish to tantalise the taste buds.

If the closest you've ever got to herbs is a dollop of mustard on roast beef or a dribble of mint sauce (out of a jar) over the lamb chop, then it is time to wake up to a whole new world of sensational aromas and flavours.

In distant times, when food was often made from a few monotonous staples and was sometimes none too fresh, herbs were used to liven up the boring tastes and to cover up the unpleasant ones. The cooks of ancient Rome and Greece became expert at using the wonderful aromatic herbs of the Mediterranean, and the good news soon spread all over Europe. Garlic came to us from Asia, chives from China, and tarragon from Russia.

By the Middle Ages, herb or 'pot' gardens abounded throughout the British Isles. Many of the plants were grown for their medical qualities, but those planted for the pot were just as important. It is simple to grow a selection of your own. Plant them near to the kitchen, not in some forgotten, distant corner of the garden, in tubs on a patio or balcony, in windowboxes or even on the kitchen windowsill.

Here are a selection of herbs that are easy to grow and store and will add a magical new dimension to your reputation, both as a gardener and a gourmet cook.

Balm Otherwise known as lemon balm, this herb is equally helpful for calming nervous tension or the anxious, nervous indigestion that so often goes with it. It is useful, too, for over-excited, or anxious children; in Spain it's considered a nursery cure-all. The leaves make a pleasant, soothing tea. It has a strong scent but a much milder flavour, so is perfect as an addition to fruit salad, jellies, custard, or even to the more delicate soups. It is best added as chopped leaves towards the end of cooling.

This is a hardy perennial which likes rich, moist soil and plenty of sun, but it will grow almost anywhere. The scent of the flowers is great for attracting bees: the ancient Greeks planted it for just this reason. Use the fresh leaves throughout the summer, but cut those you plan to dry, just before flowering.

Basil Is both tonic and calming to the nervous system – a natural tranquilliser for the frazzled nerves that lead to insomnia. If this is your problem, have a good *soupe au pistou* in the evening. Essential for any tomato dish, one of the best of all pasta sauces is *pesto*, made from basil, garlic, pine kernels and olive oil. Add it to soups, salads, fish and poultry; use with cooked vegetables like potatoes, courgettes, onions and beetroot. Never wash basil – the leaves turn black – wipe with a damp cloth and tear into small bits.

Basil really likes the southern sunshine; it is an annual in the UK. Grow in a well-drained pot in a sheltered, sunny spot. Bring it into the house in September, keep on a sunny windowsill, and you will have fresh leaves through the winter. They can be dried or frozen, but I prefer to use them to flavour a couple of bottles of olive oil.

Bay The distinctive flavour of bay leaves is an intrinsic part of the classic French *bouquet garni* – prized as much for their antiseptic properties as for their assistance to the digestion, helping to ward off gas and cramps. Tuck a bay leaf or two inside a chicken, but remove before cooking. Add them from the start, too, to fish, soups, stews and casseroles. This herb gives a subtle taste to some sweet dishes like custard and milk puddings, but the leaves should be removed when the flavour is strong enough. Pick leaves as needed and break in half before use. Never crush them, and make sure they are removed from dishes before liquidising, as very small bits may be injurious.

This slow-growing, perennial evergreen, once well established, will survive in the southern counties. It is probably best grown in pots and protected with sacking during severe weather.

Borage The old herbalists used this pretty herb as an anti-depressant. Adding the leaves and flowers to wine was reputed to make people happy and carefree. It has a slight cucumber taste which makes the leaves ideal with fish, potato salad and cottage cheese. A sprig of leaves and flowers is the perfect complement to a glass of Pimm's or cold red wine punch.

An annual which will self-seed, borage can be grown in any soil, in a sunny position. Plant at least 2 feet from the plants. Use the young leaves during summer, picking the flowers fresh as needed; but for freezing or drying, gather them when just open.

Caraway In Central Europe caraway seeds are a well-known aid to digestion; people chew a few of them before sitting down to a rich meal. They are particularly effective – like dill, which contains the same compound, carvone – for coping with wind or flatulence. Add them to potentially windy dishes, such as cabbage or beans, or make an infusion of them to soothe indigestion.

Caraway is a hardy biennial which thrives in well-drained soil in full sun. The young leaves can be added to salads, but it is the seed that you want to harvest. Cut the plants off at the base when the seeds ripen – July/August – then tie them in bunches, and hang, heads down, over a clean sheet of cotton, preferably in a dry, airy shed.

Chamomile   Insomnia, nervous indigestion and the jitters all respond to this magically calming herb, which makes one of the most pleasant of all herbal teas. Whenever ordinary tea or coffee are contra-indicated, this should be one of your first choices. It is one of the best indigestion cures, and has a good anti-inflammatory action which helps with joint problems and period pains.

A perennial which grows just about anywhere, chamomile is ideal for pots or troughs, as well as gardens. Use the fresh flowers for your tea and pick them to dry when they are in full bloom.

Chervil   Traditionally recommended for high blood pressure and thrombosis, it is also helpful in the reduction of gouty swellings and the elimination of chronic catarrh. The delicate anise flavour is best preserved by adding the leaves right at the end of the cooking time or afterwards. Use in soups, fish, salads and omelettes.

Chervil is another hardy annual which will self-seed when grown in partial shade in just about any soil. Use the fresh leaves, or collect them for freezing as they are not good for drying.

Chives   These share many of the wonderful healing properties of garlic and onions, which belong to the same family of plants. Use them, cut in thin rings, as a garnish on salads, sprinkled onto soups, or cooked with scrambled eggs and omelettes. Add the purple flowers to salads – they look great and taste even better.

A perennial which dies back in the winter, chives will grow almost anywhere, but prefer good moist soil and some sun. Perfect for pots, they do best when cut often to stimulate new growth. Trim off with scissors to within an inch of the soil. Chives don't dry well, so make sure you freeze plenty before they start to die back.

Dill   Most babies taste dill in the familiar form of gripe water – for which few plants could be more effective. Its name comes from a Saxon word meaning 'to lull', and is one of the best digestive aids. The chopped leaves are good in soups and fish dishes; added to cooked marrow, mushrooms and cabbage, they impart a delicate flavour; and they are a prime ingredient for making pickled cucumbers. The seeds are used with cabbage, fish, cheese and stews.

Dill is a hardy annual which likes well-drained soil and plenty of sun. Use the leaves before flowering, unopened flower heads for 'dill pickles' and gather the seeds as they start turning brown (the same method as for caraway).

Fennel The seeds and the feathery fronds are equally effective aids to digestion. Tea made from the crushed, dried seeds is a remedy for gas, colic or stomach cramps. It has a similar but stronger flavour than dill, and is the perfect herb for oily fish like herring and mackerel, which should be grilled on its sprigs. Sprinkle the chopped fronds on salads and vegetables and add the seeds to the liquid used for poached fish.

A hardy perennial which does well in the garden or pots, fennel needs some sun. The fresh fronds are good for freezing but not for drying.

Garlic This is the undisputed king of the healing plants. None other has enjoyed such a wide-ranging reputation as a cure for so many ailments in so many countries. Garlic has been the subject of more modern research than most of the other culinary herbs put together. It is effective in the treatment and prevention of heart disease and has a powerful effect on chest infections of all types, from colds to bronchitis. Intestinal infections respond well to this humble little bulb, as do urinary infections, rheumatism, arthritis and gout. Some studies even hint that garlic may have certain anti-cancer properties. Indeed, there are almost as many uses for garlic as there are recipes, and few savoury dishes will not be improved with a hint of this wonderful herb.

Garlic is one of the easiest, yet least grown, of all the herbs. It is an annual, produced by planting the individual cloves from a bulb. They should go in during November or March, and will be ready to gather when the leaves die back in July or August. They just need weeding, and watering in very dry weather. Leave them to dry in airy conditions, then tie on to a string and hang up in a warm, dry place.

Horseradish This belongs to the same species as watercress and shares many of its tonic and curative powers, including a strong antibiotic action. Most of us know this condiment only as made up in jars, to be eaten with roast beef. Try the fresh root grated into salad dressing, mayonnaise or cottage cheese. Add a little to natural yoghurt as an accompaniment to smoked fish.

Horseradish is a hardy herbaceous perennial which is easy to grow, but it can take over the garden. It will thrive anywhere, but for good roots, it is best to have a well-dug patch with plenty of manure. From one plant, you can propagate from root cuttings and end up with a whole bed. Plant in February and you'll be making your own sauce by the autumn. Dig up a root when you need it, but for drying or storing over winter in boxes of damp sand, lift in the autumn.

Lemon verbena With a much stronger flavour than the lemon balm, and longer lasting, this beautiful herb makes a delicious and strongly sedative tea.

A deciduous perennial which may suffer in severe winters, it does best in a sheltered spot, against a south wall, and in well-drained soil. It can grow to about 8 feet, but a pot will restrict the growth and allow the plant to be taken in during bad winters. Use the fresh leaves up to late September, but those for drying should be gathered just before flowering. Put a few dried leaves in with your bottom drawer – they keep their scent for years.

Marjoram (or Oregano) The volatile oil of this aromatic herb is powerfully sedative and, in fact, it is one of the great calmers. Use it for nerves and indigestion. It is a good remedy for chest infections, so eat lots of it during the winter months. Add it to salads, or at the end of cooking to soups, meat dishes, poultry, winter stews, vegetables and, sparingly, to cheese dishes. The wonderful aromas of Italian cooking come mainly from the wild marjoram or oregano. Wherever pizza is in the oven, or tomatoes in the pan, oregano is there too.

All the marjorams are easy to grow and will do well in pots. Sow the seeds in April, or divide established plants in late summer. They prefer light, well-drained soil and sunshine. Pick fresh shoots from spring to autumn. Sweet marjoram is the only variety that dries well; pick whole shoots with leaves and flowers.

Mint Green tea made with peppermint leaves is popular as a digestive all over the Middle East – and deservedly so. All the mints are wonderful digestive aids, which also stimulate the heart and nerves. The wise will drink this delicious tea instead of coffee for its mild lift – but not in the evening when it may be over-stimulating. In country medicine the mints have always had a reputation for being distinctly aphrodisiac!

Add sprigs to potatoes and peas while cooking; use chopped leaves when grilling veal or lamb chops, in carrots, beans and aubergines. They are surprisingly good in sweet dishes like muesli, yoghurt sauce served with dried fruit, strawberries, ice cream and drinks such as Pimm's or mint julep.

There are many varieties of mint and they all grow like weeds, thriving in any soil, but not liking too much sun. They will spread all over your garden, so grow them in an old bucket without a bottom, sunk into the ground, or in pots. Use fresh whenever possible, but pick mints for drying when the flowers are not quite fully open.

Parsley   Rich in vitamins A and C, and in iron, calcium and potassium. Herbalists value it specially for its diuretic action, and prescribe it for kidney and bladder problems; parsley tea was used in the trenches of the First World War for soldiers suffering kidney complications following dysentery. It also helps eliminate uric acid, making it useful in dealing with rheumatism and gout.

Parsley is the most used and most versatile of the culinary herbs, but none the less valuable for that. The stalks have more flavour than the leaves, so use them in stews and casseroles, marinades and stocks. The leaves may be added to egg dishes, fish, meat and poultry, salads, vegetables and many sauces.

A hardy biennial which prefers rich, damp soil and not too much sun, parsley grows well in pots and can be picked fresh for most of the year. It does not dry well, but is good for freezing.

Rosemary   It's hardly surprising that rosemary is valued for its powers of 'remembrance'; it is a powerful tonic and stimulant of the adrenal cortex. So it is valuable in states of general debility, including loss of memory, strain and nervous tension. Rosemary is also tonic and soothing to the digestive tract; try it for dyspepsia, gas and flatulence.

Most often used with roast lamb, this wonderful, pungent herb can be added to poultry, marinades, soups, stews, stuffings, vegetables and even in savoury scones. You probably haven't tried it in sweets, but it makes a tantalising lemon and rosemary sorbet!

This hardy evergreen needs light, well-drained soil, sun and shelter. Young plants will need some protection in harsh weather. Pick sprigs for use throughout the growing period, but if you want to dry this herb, gather it in just as it starts flowering.

Sage   A powerful antiseptic and healer (try it as a gargle for sore throats). It also acts as a stimulant to the central nervous system, making it a valuable tonic for convalescents or for those suffering from stress or nervous exhaustion. This herb is a good aid to digestion, particularly of fatty foods, so it is a sound idea to use it in the stuffing of roast meats and poultry. The slightly bitter taste goes well with liver, duck, goose, pork sausages and stews. The leaves should be chopped, except with fried calves' liver, when they are used whole.

These hardy, evergreen shrubs grow well in pots or in sunny, light, well-drained soil. Pick the leaves fresh when needed, but for drying gather them just before the bush flowers.

Savory Its German name means 'bean-herb' since it eases the digestion of this challenging food and benefits the entire digestive tract. It has an antiseptic action on the gut and its aphrodisiac powers are legendary – but no doubt exaggerated. The slightly peppery taste mixes well with other herbs, and is good for all bean dishes, in soups, marinades, with fish, poultry, game and pork.

The two varieties are winter and summer savory. The former has a stronger taste, so use sparingly. They both do well in pots, and like well-drained soil and sunshine. Use fresh leaves and pick shoots for drying before the plants flower.

Sweet cicely This favourite of the old herbalists is said to be relaxing, a good digestive aid, helpful for flatulence and a good expectorant.

The leaves and young fruits may be chewed – they have a slight anise flavour. The chopped leaves are good in soups and salads, also with all the root vegetables. Sprigs of the fresh plant may be added to sour fruits like rhubarb, plums, damsons, berries and currants, thus sweetening the fruit and reducing the quantity of sugar needed in cooking. The chopped leaves can be sprinkled onto fresh strawberries or gooseberries.

It will grow anywhere, but does best in damp soil and half-shade. The leaves freeze, but are not suitable for drying.

Tarragon Another of the culinary herbs which is good for the digestive system, relieving gas, flatulence and acidity. Use it to replace salt – important in the treatment of high blood pressure.

This herb, with its slightly bitter, liquorice taste, is surely one of the most important in the kitchen. Add the chopped leaves to poultry, eggs, offal, fish, shellfish, herb butter and most vegetables. Use fresh leaves through the season, but pick for freezing around midsummer. Tarragon is not good for drying, but it makes wonderful flavoured oil and vinegar.

A hardy perennial, it needs light, well-drained soil and a sunny spot. It will grow well in pots.

Thyme Thyme is a general stimulant to the body's natural resistance, with marked anti-viral and anti-bacterial activity – particularly effective in cases of flu. Thyme is also a tonic to the nervous system. Among its essential oils is thymol, a remarkably potent antiseptic; and herbalists use doses of thyme tea to treat infections not only of the respiratory system but also of the intestines and the urinary tract.

Thyme is another versatile herb which can be used in stocks, marinades, soups, meat and all game dishes. Add it to pasta, salads and vegetables and stuffings.

All varieties are hardy, evergreen perennials, which grow well in pots. They like well-drained soil and lots of sun. Use fresh shoots for cooking, but collect your thyme for drying before it flowers.

How to gather, dry and store your herbs

If you have gone to all the trouble of growing your own herbs, then it is worth making the effort to ensure you can enjoy them all year round. You are bound to have some disasters, but this is half the fun. The more you experiment, the better your results, so keep trying and you will get it right.

Picking

Leaves are best gathered for storage when at their prime. For most herbs this means just before they flower. Try to pick them early on a dry morning, and as soon as the dew is off. Unless they are very dirty, don't wash them, but when unavoidable, rinse quickly and only in cold water. Leave them to dry on a paper towel.

Flowers should be cut when they are well out but not over-mature, and should never be washed.

Seeds can be saved by leaving the plant as long as possible, then cutting off the seed head, hanging it over a newspaper and waiting for the seeds to drop.

Drying

This must be done slowly and gently. Hang your herbs in bunches, upside down, in a warm, airy and dry place, where there is little light. This will preserve both flavour and colour. The garden shed, loft, airing cupboard or garage will do, but if the weather is very wet, you may need some extra heat for outside places. Flowers are best dried in single layers on wooden trays lined with newspaper. If there is no alternative, try the slow-cook compartment, or the plate warmer of your oven, but don't let the temperature go above 90°F (32°C). Leaves are ready to store when they feel brittle, flowers when they are papery.

Some people even use a microwave: three minutes or so is enough for most leaves, but you can keep trying till they become brittle.

Storing

All dried herbs must be kept in airtight containers. Dark glass or pottery jars are best, as both air and light will spoil the flavour.

Freezing

Many of the herbs can be frozen. There is no need to blanch, just put them into double polythene bags, which stops the strong aromas from tainting other food, then place in the freezer. My favourite trick with herbs like parsley, dill, fennel and chives, is to chop the leaves, sprinkle a teaspoonful into each compartment of an ice cube tray, add water and freeze. Store the cubes in large double bags, and just add them to stews, soups or other dishes.

Garlic

A few years ago, one of those strange coincidences that happen in life turned me into a garlic freak. Within the space of one week, three separate patients told me that their doctors were puzzled by changes in the behaviour of their blood samples. They had all consulted me with different problems, but all had heart or circulatory problems, and the three of them were taking anti-coagulant drugs to 'thin' the blood, and all had had their dose of medication reduced.

Why did I find this news so exciting? Because the only treatment that I had prescribed, which was the same for all of them, was large doses of garlic.

Since my student days I had been taught the value of this remarkable plant, but now I became an avid reader of anything I could find about it.

In ancient Egypt, Greece and Rome, and in Britain during the Middle Ages and up to the end of the last century, garlic was the most widely used of all medicinal plants. Bronchitis, catarrh, sore throats, tonsillitis, asthma, indigestion, constipation, diarrhoea and even athlete's foot, can all be helped by this powerful little bulb. It has long been known that garlic has a broad anti-bacterial effect – first proved scientifically by Louis Pasteur in 1858; that it can destroy fungi; and that it is a useful antidote to some poisons, especially alcohol and heavy metals.

As a home remedy, try a crushed clove, mixed with a dessertspoon of honey, a squeeze of lemon juice, and dissolved in a cup of hot water. It's just the thing to take, three times a day, for catarrh, bronchitis and sinus problems.

For indigestion, constipation and mild stomach upsets, crush one clove of garlic into a cup of warm milk and drink after meals. If you suffer from cystitis or other urinary infections, then crush a clove into a small carton of natural yoghurt, and make sure that you eat one pot each morning and evening.

These are just some of the traditional uses for garlic, but by far the most exciting development in the history of this plant is the latest research into its powerful effect on the heart and circulation.

Garlic has the unique ability to both prevent, and treat, some of the factors which are linked to heart disease. Scientists who study the distribution of illnesses in different populations, know that in those countries where large quantities are eaten there is a lower rate of death from heart attacks. This is despite the fact that in many of these countries there is just as much smoking and drinking as there is in the UK. We have the lowest consumption of garlic in Europe, and the highest rate of premature death from heart disease.

Some 180,000 people die from heart disease each year in the UK – that's the population of Swansea – whilst half a million suffer a heart attack. The sulphur compound, allicin, released when garlic is crushed, both encourages the elimination of cholesterol from the body, and reduces the quantity of the unhealthy fats which are produced by the liver. In healthy volunteers, on fatty diets, it has been shown to reduce the level of cholesterol in the blood by up to 15 per cent.

At the Second International Garlic Symposium in Berlin, some of the most exciting work presented was about reduction of blood cholesterol, high blood pressure and blood clots, the three most important factors involved in heart disease and strokes.

Dr Mader described a study by thirty GPs of 261 patients with raised cholesterol. This was a randomised, double blind trial in which half the patients were given a placebo and half garlic in the form of standardised Kwai garlic tablets.

No dietary advice was included in the treatment and the cholesterol was measured after each four-week period for a total of sixteen weeks. Both groups showed an initial reduction in cholesterol, but as the study progressed the placebo group remained steady, whilst the garlic group reduced their cholesterol by an average of 12 per cent.

Cholesterol is essential to the body, but problems can arise if you have too much in your blood. If your level is higher than it should be – simple tests are now widely available – your doctor will advise a healthier diet and lifestyle: stop smoking, take more exercise, eat less saturated fat and more fibre. We now know that taking garlic can help lower the amount of 'bad' LDL-cholesterol and raise the level of the 'good' HDL-cholesterol. It also makes blood less likely to clot, improves circulation and helps lower moderately raised blood pressure.

Garlic research is being done all round the world and I'm delighted that the orthodox medics are accepting the great role that this plant has to play in the prevention and treatment of disease.

A report in the *British Medical Journal* confirms the benefits of garlic in heart disease, but emphasises the importance of using preparations containing adequate amounts of the active principle, allicin, which may not be present in extracts or oils made by steam distillation.

Work in the eye hospital at Aachen University, in the Transfusion

Institute at the University of Saarland, and the University of Munich, now provides clear evidence that garlic dilates blood vessels and reduces the stickiness of the blood.

As if all this research were not surprising enough, garlic also has protective properties against cancer. Professor Kourounakis, from Greece, and Professor Wargovich, from the University of Texas, are both working in this field. The Greeks have investigated the way in which garlic can destroy chemicals called 'free radicals'. They are highly destructive and can initiate the production of cancerous cells in the body. Kourounakis told me that their first studies have been so impressive that exciting follow-up work is already in progress. Wargovich is looking at a wide range of natural compounds, and studying their protective effect against cancer-inducing chemicals. Both before and after exposure to the toxic compounds, garlic reduced, and in some cases, prevented the development of some experimental cancers.

So, what's the best way to get your garlic? It's not all the same and the quality varies depending on the soil in which it's grown. The best is grown organically in China and gives a rich yield of the vital sulphur compound, allicin, which is destroyed by crushing or cooking. If you don't fancy munching a raw clove a day, you can take a garlic supplement. But which to choose?

Look for whole, dried garlic powder in tablets which retain the goodness of the fresh clove. There must be a high proportion of allicin, and to ensure the effective dose, the product should be standardised – each pill in each batch contains an exact dose. Two tablets of Kwai garlic, taken three times daily, is the same as a medium, fresh, high quality clove. The special coating on the pills means that both taste and smell are controlled and no one will complain!

I am pleased that after twenty-five years of advising anyone who would listen to add garlic to their diet, science is proving the 'old wives' to be right.

Guarana – the healing herb from the rain forest

We have a lot to learn about the medicinal value of plants from the Indians in Brazil.

'If we continue to destroy the rain forest, we will be depriving mankind of potential medical benefits which are beyond our wildest dreams. Cures for cancer, AIDS, lupus, leukaemia and who knows what else, could be going up in smoke as thousands of plants are being wiped off the face of the Earth.'

These were the opening words from ethnobotanist, Dr Walter Accorsi, Professor of Botany at São Paulo University, when we met in Brazil. He is the founder of the Brazilian Botanical Society and

Director of the Medicinal Plant Research Laboratory at the university, and a passionate worker for the protection of the rain forest flora.

Is it too late? Thanks to the efforts of a handful of far-sighted people, hopefully not. One of these is a young Englishman, Grahame Lewis, who went to Brazil for a holiday, lived for two years on a remote island and fell under the spell of the Amazon, its people, and its plants. He was determined to try to help, so began importing some of the Indian herbal medicines to England. I went with him to the rain forest to find out more about one of the most effective of all the traditional remedies, guarana.

Our journey took us on a sixteen-hour flight to the town of Manaus, at the Amazon basin, and then by boat, down the river to the small village of Maues, thirty hours of gentle meandering on the Amazon itself, and then through a maze of smaller tributaries. No matter what you have read, heard or seen about the Amazon and the rain forest, nothing prepares you for the first sights, sounds and smells. The majesty of a waterway, so wide that in places you cannot see either bank. Pink, freshwater dolphins playing around the boat; endless tracts of dense, impenetrable jungle, with just the odd hut or small settlement, built on stilts along the water's edge; tiny dugout canoes, barely above the water; flocks of screeching parrots, heron and vultures; as night falls, the total silence and darkness, and with it clouds of angry mosquitoes.

The tiny settlement of Maues is stuck in a time warp. The clocks seem to have stopped around the 1920s. But here there is a glimmer of hope. Maues is the centre of the guarana industry – an industry which is a marriage of tribal wisdom, idealism and modern pharmacology.

First discovered by the Maué-saterés tribe, guarana has been used for thousands of years as a tonic and stimulant. So valuable was it to the tribesmen, that this plant was a form of currency throughout the rain forests. The earliest reports of the value of guarana came from a missionary called Betendorf. The Maué-saterés were by far the sturdiest and healthiest tribe which he found during his travels in the forest. In 1669 he wrote of the way in which the Indians used the plant to help them cope with the extreme heat, to carry them through long journeys, to suppress the appetite and to relieve headaches, fevers and cramp.

This extraordinary plant gets its name from a native word which means 'secret eyes'. If you are ever fortunate enough to see it growing you'll know why. The fruit of this luxuriant shrub hangs in great bunches, like bright red grapes. The red pods split to reveal chestnut-brown seeds with a white round middle. As you walk in the forest they are like a million eyes staring out at you.

I drove in an open truck, during a tropical thunderstorm, through one of the largest plantations in the Amazon – as big as Guernsey. There, the seeds are harvested and processed as they have been for generations.

Nothing much has changed since the 17th century. We found small communities of Indians, two or three families, still producing guarana in the original way. But this is now an organised industry. The berries are collected, soaked to remove the outer husks, then washed, dried, crushed and roasted in giant clay dishes made from river mud, straw and ashes. Finally they are ground with a giant wooden pestle and mortar, rolled into sticks of paste and baked hard over a smoke fire.

Traditionally, the day starts with a cup of guarana tea. It is made by grating the end of the bread-stick into boiling water. The grater is the bone-hard, rough palate of an Amazonian fish, the pirarucu. I ate the fish, which was wonderful, and shared the tea with the local Indians.

As well as producing this traditional form of the herb, more convenient products, like capsules and dry powder, are made for export all over South America, and now even to Great Britain. The national soft drink in Brazil is not the universal 'Coke', but one made from the guarana seed. So what is it that makes this plant so valuable to man?

One of the main constituents of guarana is a chemical called guaranine. This is similar in structure to caffeine, which would explain the tonic and stimulating effects. There have been attempts to isolate the active principle and use it as a medicine. But, as so often happens, the native wisdom has been proved right. The Indians only ever use the whole seed and this works without side effects. Although the caffeine-like properties are present, in combination with the other ingredients in the plant it has a gentle and sustained effect.

The tannin content is relatively high, too, and this explains why guarana is so good for the treatment of diarrhoea and digestive problems. What's more, there are potent saponins, similar to those found in ginseng. It is these that balance the stimulation produced by the guaranine. I am certain that guarana tea is a good substitute for tea and coffee. It will provide that lift which we have come to expect, but in a much gentler and longer lasting way. It could be useful for those who need to avoid caffeine, those with migraine or high blood pressure, but who still feel like a light stimulant at some time during the day.

The Indians say that guarana prevents and combats fatigue, stimulates brain function, aids concentration, relieves headache and menstrual pain, helps the body get rid of water, combats the discomfort of extreme heat, speeds recovery after illness and reduces appetite.

So, who can benefit from these 'secret eyes' from the jungle? Anyone under stress or pressure – exams, interviews, work, social functions – as well as people who are ill, convalescents and nursing mothers. I have found it particularly valuable, too, for my patients with ME, a condition that needs a source of energy which is more than short-term stimulation.

Youngsters 'out on the town' have discovered that guarana is the ideal way to boost their energy for nights of disco dancing and partying – and it's legal!

Science is uncovering some of the mysteries of the rain forest plants. Guarana has uses as a tonic and stimulant; it is a mild diuretic and can help treat stomach upsets; it reduces temperature, controls hunger, overcomes fatigue and is a safe mild anti-depressant. According to Professor Accorsi, the herb lapacho is equally exciting. Long used by the Indians as a treatment for skin problems and scars, it now seems that it may have some anti-cancer action. As a result of some observational studies at his Institute, scientists in America, Japan and Brazil are now working on the chemical actions of this plant. Accorsi stresses that this work is at an early stage, and it could be years before there is a usable body of evidence.

It may not be long before many of the other plants which could alleviate man's suffering vanish in the face of man's greed. Men of vision, like Grahame Lewis and his partners in the Rio Trading Company, are fighting to protect the heritage of the rain forest Indians and bring us the benefits of their herbs such as guarana and lapacho.

Finding your way round the vitamin maze

Edwina Currie was right all along. If she had stayed at the Department of Health we might have had some healthy changes in the government's eating advice a lot sooner.

It has taken the Committee on Medical Aspects of Food Policy (COMA), four years to produce its report on how we should be improving our National Diet. Four years to come to the same conclusions that many experts have been advising, around the world, since the mid-1970s.

But here it is at last: 210 pages of complex charts and tables which your GP will find confusing, you will find incomprehensible and the giant food manufacturers will find a boon – they'll be able to blind you with even more science on the labels.

Here is the essence of the 'Food Revolution'.

Eat less fat, less sugar, less salt, less meat and less refined carbohydrates. Eat more fresh fruit, vegetables and salads, more wholegrain cereals, beans, pulses, fish and poultry.

Sounds familiar? It is probably pretty close to granny's advice. And if you take your holidays in Spain, Portugal, Italy, Greece or the south of France, it is the basis of the 'Mediterranean Diet' which you enjoyed so much, and which helps to keep their levels of heart disease and some types of cancer so much lower than those in the UK.

The new report has radically changed the system for calculating how much of each nutrient we need, and this is going to take some getting used to.

The RDA – recommended daily amount – which has been with us for years, is now replaced by the RNI – reference nutrient intake – the quantity of a nutrient which is sufficient for 97 per cent of the population.

Some of the figures have gone down, some up, and for the first time the COMA report lists RNIs for nutrients which complementary practitioners have advised for years.

There are variations for age, sex, pregnancy and breast feeding; and of course those with certain specific diseases need extra nutrients. But, for the average man or woman aged 19-49, here is a guide to what you should be getting, and how the new figures compare with the old.

	Old RDA		New RNI	
	Female	Male	Female	Male
protein	54 g	66 g	45 g	55 g
energy	2150 kcal	2900 kcal	1940 kcal	2250 kcal
calcium	500 mg	500 mg	700 mg	700 mg
iron	12 mg	10 mg	14.8 mg	8.7 mg
zinc	NIL	NIL	7 mg	9.5 mg
copper	NIL	NIL	1.2 mg	1.2 mg
salt	9 g	9 g	4 g	4 g
potassium	NIL	NIL	3500 mg	3500 mg
magnesium	NIL	NIL	270 mg	300 mg
phosphorus	NIL	NIL	540 mg	540 mg
Vitamins				
A	750 μg[1]	750 μg	600 μg	700 μg
C	30 mg	30 mg	40 mg	40 mg
D	10 μg	10 μg	Not if exposed to sun	
E	NIL	NIL	5 mg	7 mg
B1	0.9 mg	1 mg	0.8 mg	1 mg
B2	1.3 mg	1.6 mg	1.1 mg	1.3 mg
Niacin	15 mg	18 mg	12.8 mg	16.8 mg
B6	NIL	NIL	1.2 mg	1.4 mg
B12	NIL	NIL	1.5 μg	1.5 μg
Folic acid	NIL	NIL	200 μg	200 μg

[1] 1 μg (microgram) equals one-thousandth of a milligram.

You can see what I mean about confusing. These figures don't say much to the average shopper pushing a trolley round the supermarket. They get even more meaningless when you are faced by rows and rows of vitamin pills on the shelves of the health store. What's more, the health shop assistants do not seem to know much about them either, although family owned local shops tend to be run by enthusiasts who make a real effort to be well informed.

I always ask my patients to bring any supplements they are taking when they come to see me. Lots of them turn up with plastic bagsful! This really upsets me, as they are certainly spending too much money, and some of the vitamins and minerals can be dangerous if taken in high doses.

Another concern is the obsession which so many women have for calorie counting.

Calories are not the be-all and end-all of healthy eating. The vital factor is how those calories are obtained. You can have 90 calories from a healthy banana or an unhealthy chocolate digestive biscuit; 130 calories from 4 oz of nourishing coleslaw or 1 oz of chocolates; 180 calories from 2 oz of protein- and calcium-rich Dutch Edam or 1 oz of salted peanuts; 100 calories from two full-of-vitality apples or one mini-Mars bar; 200 calories from half an avocado – bursting with protective vitamin E – or one small chocolate cream-cake – bursting with tooth-destroying sugar!

Calories are a useful but rough guide to your daily food intake, but fewer calories from nutritionally poor food will be infinitely less healthy than a few more in a diet made up from nature's storehouse of essential goodies.

If you are about to embark on yet another binge of calorie counting, or your fourth go this year at a very low-calorie, meal replacement diet, take a look at this chart to see what your calorie needs are. COMA urges us all to increase our energy expenditure, rather than reduce consumption below the advised levels. It believes that such an increase for 'many people over the age of 1 year, would be desirable for health'.

A strict diet for a week or two, just for that special occasion, is one thing, but long-term calorie reduction without sound nutritional advice, can be a recipe for illness, not thinness.

Average Daily Calorie Needs

Age	Male	Female
1–3 years	1230	1165
4–6	1715	1545
7–10	1970	1740
11–14	2220	1845

15–18	2755	2110
19–49	2550	1940
50–59	2550	1900
60–64	2380	1900
65–74	2330	1900
75+	2100	1810

The COMA advice on calories is to get more of your energy from complex carbohydrates – bread, potatoes, rice, pasta, beans and pulses – and less from fats and refined sugars. If we all made this simple and money-saving change, the nation's health would improve very quickly.

I am most concerned about COMA's recommendations for vitamins and minerals. Despite the fact that it does now recognise the importance of vitamin E and some of the minerals, the report makes no allowance for the huge variations in the actual nutrient content in today's foods. Intensive growing methods, transporting, storage, freshness and handling, can all reduce the level of vitamins. And that's before you even buy them, take them home and cook them. The theoretical vitamin content of what ends up on your plate is often a great deal more than the reality of what you put into your mouth.

There is a difference between what you need to avoid getting ill and the amounts of vitamins and minerals which will keep you in peak condition. Here then is a list of what some of the vitamins do, and how much you have to eat to more than cover the new guidelines.

Vitamin A Essential for growth, skin, night and colour vision. All you need for a day is contained in 5 g of liver, 40 g of old carrots, 70 g of spinach, butter or margarine, or 120 g of broccoli with 60 g of cheddar cheese in a sauce.

Vitamin C Prevents scurvy, aids wound healing and iron absorption, and is a vital and protective antioxidant. The daily dose is in a dessertspoon of blackcurrant, a lemon, half a green pepper, an orange, half a large grapefruit, a kiwi fruit, or 90 g raw red cabbage.

Vitamin D Essential for bone formation as it is part of the calcium absorption system. Lack of this vitamin causes rickets in children and bone disorders in adults. The action of ultraviolet light on the skin produces vitamin D. For this reason, the report has not set a daily quantity since it maintains that few UK residents are short of it. The exceptions are the elderly and other groups who get little fresh air and daylight exposure. The Asian community is often at risk due to traditional clothing, diet and lifestyle.

The 10 μg that is essential will be obtained from 1 teaspoon of cod liver oil, 45 g of herring or kipper, 55 g mackerel, 80 g canned salmon or tuna, or 135 g canned sardines. Eggs and margarine, too, are fair sources.

Vitamin B1, Thiamin   The main function is during the conversion of carbohydrates into energy. If you live on a high starch diet – some vegetarians do – or where there is an excessive consumption of alcohol, the need for B1 increases. Your daily dose can be had from 60 g cod roe, 70 g wheatgerm or 100 g brazil or peanuts. Oatmeal, bacon, pork, offal and bread, too, are all good sources.

Vitamin B2, Riboflavin   Vital for growth and for the skin and mucous membranes. The 1.3 g you need will come from six eggs, 1½ pints of milk, 65 g of liver or kidney, or 250 g cheddar. Beef, mackerel, almonds, cereals and poultry are also good sources.

Vitamin B6, Pyridoxine   Previously there were no minimum requirements for this vitamin, which is essential for growth. Many women have found it helpful in the treatment of the symptoms of PMS, and it may overcome some of the side-effects of the Pill. Fish, meat, liver and cheese are good sources. A large banana and half an avocado will provide the daily dose. A portion of cod, salmon or a grilled herring will give you nearly all you need.

Folic acid   Vital during growth and development. Studies now show us that some birth defects may be related to a low intake, so there is now a minimum requirement for the first time. The best sources are dark green vegetables, liver, kidney, nuts, wholemeal bread and wholegrain cereals. The RNI is 200 μg, an average portion of lamb's liver supplies 250 μg, spinach 140 μg, kidney beans, frozen peas, chickpeas and raw red cabbage all around 75 μg.

Still confused? I'm not surprised. The burning question most people ask is, 'Do I need to take extra vitamins?' The theoretical answer is no, not if you are eating a well-balanced diet, and using a wide variety of foods.

In fact, few people manage to do this, and even fewer persuade their partners or children to do it. Pressures of time, working couples, no school meals, and the relentless march of the fast food industry, all make it more difficult.

So you dash to the chemist or health store to pick up a pot of pills, and by the time you have read the umpteenth label, you're more muddled than ever. Do you choose a multivitamin, six individual bottles, mega-dose, slow release, vegetarian capsules, tablets made without gluten, yeast, colourings or sugars, a brand with seventy different ingredients, one with five or, like so many shoppers, do you leave empty handed?

Even worse, you may waste a lot of your hard-earned cash on supplements you don't need, and which may do more harm than good. Single vitamins and minerals certainly have a place, but as a general rule, they are best taken (certainly the high dose ones) on the advice of your practitioner. If you mix and match yourself, you may find that the products overlap and you get more than you bargained for of some nutrients.

More than ten times the basic need of Vitamin A, taken over long periods, can cause liver and bone damage. Over 3300 μg must not be taken during pregnancy as there is a risk of birth defects. Taking a multivitamin, together with a separate A pill, can easily supply this amount, and that's before you get any from your food.

Doses of B6 in excess of 2 g per day can cause nerve damage, and in some sensitive subjects, symptoms have occurred at intakes as low as 50 mg.

Do not take huge amounts of vitamin C without advice, as more than 1 g a day has been known to cause diarrhoea and to increase the risk of kidney stones in susceptible people.

Vitamin D at ten times the daily need can be very toxic to children, and twenty-five times is dangerous for adults. Don't give more than a teaspoon of cod liver oil to the kids each day, or exceed this amount during pregnancy.

Natural health insurance, in the form of an inexpensive, well-formulated multivitamin and mineral pill can be a good idea. It will make up for the missed meal, the extra demands of a stressful life, the vitamin losses during storage, transport and cooking, and it will help after illness.

So, what do you look for on the label, and how do you choose which supplement to buy? When do you and the family need to take extra nutrients? Are there special times when they should be avoided, or when you should increase your intake?

Do read the labels carefully. Avoid pills with artificial colours, flavours and preservatives. Watch out for added sugar or sweeteners. Many children especially those with asthma, eczema or other allergy problems, and those who are hyperactive, react badly to many of the food chemicals.

On the other hand, some manufacturers are cashing in on the 'allergy' area, and making expensive products which are free of gluten, yeast, egg, milk, and everything else. Unless you know that you are allergic to these, and comparatively few people are, there is no need to go to these lengths.

Most of us are unlikely to need more than a good general multivitamin and mineral supplement. Choose those with substantial levels of the main nutrients, rather than huge lists of things you've never heard of. Adult formulations are not normally suitable for children from 2–10, who should be given the relevant products. Under 2s should only get vitamins on professional advice.

Single supplements have a place in the treatment and prevention of some conditions. Extra vitamin C as protection against colds and infections during the winter; B6, zinc and evening primrose oil for PMS and other menstrual problems; calcium for osteoporosis; beta-carotene and evening primrose oil for skin conditions; folic acid, calcium, fish oil (not fish liver oil) and multivitamins, before and during pregnancy; calcium and multivitamins when breast feeding; calcium and vitamin D for the prevention of osteoporosis (start around the mid-40s); calcium, vitamin D and multivitamins for the over 60s; extra B complex at times of stress; vitamins E, C and multivit before surgery; multivit and extra C and iron when you are dieting.

High doses of single vitamins should not be taken without advice as some of them can be toxic. There is little evidence that slow-release vitamins are that much better for you, though they can be a lot more expensive.

Some vitamins will interfere with certain forms of medication, so if you are taking prescribed medicines, do check with your doctor before starting to dose yourself. There are some forms of cancer which grow more quickly if you take extra vitamins, and some which will benefit from them, so here again you *must* speak with your consultant before taking anything other than he has prescribed.

It is, generally, daft to seek certain essentials from pills. Fibre is a good example. One brand of multivitamins labelled 'Fibre Rich' costs nearly £5 for 28 days' supply, and provides less than 5 per cent of the daily need for fibre. One hundred tablets of oat bran cost more than £3 and the dose is nine pills daily. You would get more fibre, and lots of other nutrients, from a bowl of porridge.

The family pack

Multivitamins for the over 10s in your family. My best buys are Genesis from Wassen, and Vitalia's Multivitamins with minerals and extra iron. Both carry clear labels, are simple to take, one-a-day and are good value.

Healthcraft's or Nature's Aid B complex are both very good.

The best of the B6 supplements is FSC, which is a pure and good-value preparation.

Nature's Aid vitamin C 500 mg is one of the best, as it contains added rosehip, acerola cherry and bioflavinoids – an essential part of the C complex which you do not get from pure ascorbic acid.

To protect the bones, the best of the calcium supplements is

Porosis D from Cedar Health. It is not cheap, but contains the trace mineral boron, as well as calcium and vitamin D.

There are now lots of evening primrose oil products on the market. I still prefer Efamol, and in particular the Efamol Marine, which includes fish oils. Most of the research has been done with this brand, and although there are cheaper versions, this would be my choice.

All these products are available from health stores and good chemists. You can buy cheaper and much more expensive ones, but these represent the best quality and value combined. Sometimes you get what you pay for, but in the vitamin maze, you often don't.

Don't be fooled into thinking that it won't matter what you eat as long as you take a pill. This is not true. Vitamin supplements are just that, a supplement to healthy eating. If money is the prime consideration, and your budget is stretched to the limit, add £4 to your shopping instead of spending it on pills, and you can buy a lot of extra nutrition for mum, dad and the two children!

Use the following chart as a handy guide when you go to the local health food store. It will give you the information you need when buying vitamin and mineral supplements for the family. The basic need for each group of people as a health insurance policy is shown in the following table.

Who	What	How much
2–10 years	children's multivitamin	as directed
	extra C	200 mg
11–19	multivitamin	as directed
	C	300 mg
19–50 male	multivitamin	as directed
	C	500 mg
smoker	selenium ACE	as directed
drinker	B complex	as directed
19–50 female	multivitamin	as directed
	minerals + iron	as directed
	C	500 mg
	calcium	250 mg
	folic acid	100 μg
smoker	as above	
drinker	as above	
pregnant	calcium	500 mg
	folic acid	200 μg
	C	1000 mg
	beta-carotene	as directed

lactating	calcium	750 mg
	folic acid	200 μg
	C	1000 mg
	beta-carotene	as directed
50+ male	multivitamin	as directed
	C	1000 mg
	zinc	15 mg
	B complex	as directed
	fish oil	as directed
50+ female	multivitamin	as directed
	C	1000 mg
	B complex	as directed
	calcium + vitamin D	as directed
	Efamol Marine	1500 mg

One of the best comments on vitamins came from Charlton Heston. He told me, over a healthy breakfast, that he takes a multivitamin each day. When I asked him about the American obsession with huge, mega-dose pills, he replied: 'Michael, Americans have the most expensive urine in the world!'

Understanding minerals

There are minerals which your body needs, some in tiny amounts, others in intermediate amounts, and a few in tiny traces. They are all essential, and missing out on any, even the trace minerals, can make the difference between health and sickness. For example, a breast-feeding mum needs 1250 mg of calcium each day, but only 15 mg of iron, and 75 μg of selenium.

These magic minerals are nearly always ignored when investigating health problems. Except for the obvious iron and maybe calcium, most doctors couldn't tell you what they are, let alone what they do. The plain fact is that they are often a key factor in the cause of illness, and the addition of a simple supplement of the missing substances can produce dramatic improvements.

Because of modern intensive farming methods, soil that has been artificially fertilised and had the same crop grown on it for years may have its natural stores of the trace elements depleted. The crops and the animals fed on them may then contain less than we need. The same is true for cereals, fruits and vegetables.

Last year, the Department of Health published its long-awaited new guidelines for nutrition. The following table gives the daily reference nutrient intake for the average man and woman, for the minerals which are essential for life. There are others which play an important role in the way our bodies work, but for which the

Department has not established minimum daily requirements. Note especially that there are risks in taking too much of some of these minerals, and maximum safe intake levels have been advised. (See individual listings.)

New RNI

	Female	Male
calcium	700 mg	700 mg
iron	14.8 mg	8.7 mg
zinc	7 mg	9.5 mg
copper	1.2 mg	1.2 mg
sodium	4.0 mg	4.0 mg
potassium	3500 mg	3500 mg
magnesium	270 mg	300 mg
phosphorus	540 mg	540 mg
chloride	2500 mg	2500 mg
selenium	60 μg	75 μg
iodine	140 μg	140 μg

Two of the trace minerals are of special interest to me as they are the ones that can be used with dramatic effect and are often lacking in our diets.

Zinc   Vital for growth, healthy sex organs, reproduction, insulin production and natural resistance. Lack of zinc can lead to weight loss, skin diseases, ulcers and acne, lower sex-drive, loss of taste and smell, and brittle nails. Too much will reduce the copper in the body. The best places to find it are lamb, liver, steak, garlic, ginger-root, brazil nuts, pumpkin seeds, oysters, eggs, sardines, oats, crab, almonds and chicken.

Zinc deficiency can be a factor in so many conditions that I am always on the look-out for this mineral. You are more likely to have too little if you are a strict vegetarian, are constantly on weight reducing diets or if you are into some extreme food fad like macrobiotics.

Pre-menstrual tension and post-natal depression are two conditions which almost always respond well to small doses of extra zinc – around 15 mg each day. Not surprisingly, people with anorexia nervosa – the slimmer's disease – have very low levels of zinc. So taking a zinc supplement, together with all the other therapies used to treat this awful illness, can really help.

A lack of zinc may be linked to hyperactivity in children, and this could even start during pregnancy if mum is a bit low on her own intake. It will help with teenage acne, too, so make sure that you and your family get plenty of the right foods. But don't eat vast quantities of bran, as this can stop the zinc from being absorbed by the body.

Selenium   Is part of the self-defence system and is also important for cholesterol control. Deficiency may lead to low resistance, heart disease and skin problems. You will find most in wholemeal bread made from imported flour, butter, oily fish, liver, kidney and brazil nuts.

Back in the 1970s doctors in China studied 9000 young men in areas known to have very little selenium in the soil. Some were given a real pill containing tiny amounts of selenium, others a fake pill. The reduction in the rate of a heart disease common in China was so dramatic among those given the real medicine that the trial was stopped and all the men given the trace element.

We now know that selenium works together with vitamin E as an antioxidant, which attacks the free radicals that do so much damage to the body's cells. For this reason it seems a key factor in protection against high blood pressure, strokes and heart attacks.

But perhaps the most exciting function of selenium is its apparent ability to protect the body from cancer. American studies have shown that where the soil is richest in this seemingly insignificant substance, the number of people who get cancer is 20 per cent lower than in parts of the country which have soil poor in selenium.

You only need to take 100 *micro*grams a day to make sure that your body never gets short of this vital element.

Here is a selection of some of the other vital magic minerals:

Germanium   The most recently 'discovered' of the trace elements. Research in Japan has found that it is essential for life. It is known to protect plants from infection, improve their growth rate and strengthen them in general. It seems that its effect comes from the mineral's ability to act as a scavenger of free radicals – those unwanted oxygen molecules that cause oxidation – so increasing the oxygen available to the blood.

This is an abundant mineral in nature, and the average diet will give you around 1 mg a day. Doses of 50–250 mg daily, for long periods, four to eighteen months, can be seriously harmful, and may even cause death. Research is still in its infancy, so don't believe all the extravagant claims made for the germanium pills now on the market. Some of the germanium products have been withdrawn from sale, and I never advise anyone to use this mineral as a supplement.

Iron Combines with oxygen to make haemoglobin, the red colouring of the blood. This transports the air you breathe to every cell of the body. Without enough of it you will get anaemia, fatigue, depression, palpitations, and you will look pale. Too much can lower your natural resistance and also cause insomnia, tiredness and depression. Kelp (seaweed), molasses, pig's liver, beef, pilchards, kidney beans, brazil nuts, dates, raisins, lentils, peanuts, chicken, soya beans and peas are good sources of iron.

A good portion of liver, chili con carne, any game meats or beef, with green veg, peas or dried beans, will provide your daily need. Black pudding, oily fish such as pilchards, herrings and sardines, shellfish, chickpeas and kidney beans, are good sources. Spinach is not much use for iron as it contains oxalic acid which prevents it from being absorbed. The tannin in tea also interferes with iron absorption and is a factor in anaemia, especially in elderly people, whose diet may be poor and who drink lots of strong tea. Bran and cereals can cause problems, too, but vitamin C taken at the same time as cereals improves the iron uptake.

Copper Works with iron to make red blood corpuscles, important for bone formation, breakdown of cholesterol and the skin pigment melanin. A deficiency can lead to anaemia, hair problems, raised cholesterol and dry skin. Too much can be a cause of zinc deficiency. Get your daily dose from oysters, nuts, beef, liver, lamb, butter, barley and olive oil.

Calcium A vital mineral for the formation and continuing strength of bones. This is of even greater importance during pregnancy and breast feeding, and for children and teenagers. In later life women are at risk of osteoporosis (brittle bone disease), which is caused by a combination of too little calcium in the diet and poor absorption.

The time to do something positive about protecting bones is in childhood. A diet which contains lots of calcium-rich foods is the first step. Encourage children to be active, play sport and enjoy plenty of fresh air and sunshine. As you get older, these all become even more important. Pregnant and nursing mothers need to have a good store of calcium, and to take extra care of their own eating habits. When you reach your 30s make a super effort to keep up some sort of regular exercise regime. It should be weight bearing, to strengthen the bones, like tennis, dancing, keep fit classes or walking.

The menopause is a crucial period. All the symptoms are only too obvious. All, that is, except those of our secret enemy. Consider the question of Hormone Replacement Therapy (HRT) and take some extra calcium as a supplement.

Some of the things which interfere with your ability to absorb calcium are: eating too much bran; drinking large quantities of tea and alcohol; having your ovaries removed or an early menopause – before 46; having thyroid problems; and undergoing long term treatment with steroids, anti-convulsants or some of the diuretics (water pills). Furthermore, sugar, salt and smoking can all have an adverse effect.

A glass of milk, a carton of yoghurt and 2 ounces of cheese will provide the 1000 mg of calcium you need each day. Do use the low fat versions and eat plenty of tinned sardines (with the bones), lots of greens and dried fruit, nuts, beans, good bread and plenty of watercress and parsley. Your body needs sunlight to make vitamin D, without which it can't absorb the calcium, so get into the great outdoors.

Iodine   Is essential for the proper working of the thyroid gland. This produces hormones which control many of the body's functions. It also gives some degree of protection against radiation damage to the thyroid. Lack of iodine will cause lethargy, skin thickening, hair loss, growth problems and goitre. Too much may cause overactivity of the thyroid. Seaweed and sea fish are the only dependable sources. But beware of taking too much of the kelp supplements. These can be high in iodine – few of them are standardised – and may *cause* thyroid problems.

Manganese   Needed for the formation of a number of enzymes, bone formation, muscle action and fertility. A lack of it may cause bone and disc problems and high blood sugar. It's found in all whole grain cereals, nuts and tea – one cup provides nearly half the daily requirement!

Phosphorus   Is a vital mineral for bone formation and as a constituent of cells. It is present in almost all foods except fats and sugars, but those rich in calcium are the best sources. Lack of phosphorus is rare and only caused by some of the antacid drugs used for the treatment of digestive problems.

Potassium   Is essential for the proper functioning of all cells and nervous tissue. It exists in all foods except oils, fats and sugars, but can be lost into the cooking water of vegetables, so use vegetable water for soups and stews. Pills that increase the passing of urine can cause a loss of this mineral, and the risk is higher in older people who may eat less of the important foods. Most doctors prescribe the mineral with such diuretic drugs.

Boron There is little scientific evidence about the need for this mineral. It is thought to be part of the bone-forming complex. Since it is not toxic in small doses, I advise it as an aid to combating osteoporosis.

Taking mineral supplements

There are many supplements of single minerals, mineral combinations and minerals with vitamins, on the shelves in supermarkets, chemists and health stores. The choice is bewildering so that knowing which to take, if any, is like finding your way through a maze.

If your diet is a good, varied mixture of the main food groups, you are not likely to need mineral pills unless you have a particular health problem. There are certain situations when a supplement is indicated, so here is my selection of the best combination of quality and value for money:

Selenium-ACE, by Wassen, as an all-round antioxidant formulation, taken as a regular health insurance, is excellent. It provides all your needs of selenium, most of the vitamin A, more than you require of C and a significant level of E, in a convenient one-a-day tablet.

Ultra Zinc, by Power Health, supplying over twice the needed amount, one-a-day tablets. Good for poor appetite and as a regular supplement for anyone who is always catching cold.

Holland & Barrett High Potency Vitamins and Minerals for Vegetarians are good value, and provide significant amounts of minerals, together with vitamins, for the veggie in your family. Any restricted diet may lead to deficiency, so this is another good insurance.

Porosis-D, from Cedar Health, is without doubt the best of the calcium supplements: a well-balanced combination of calcium and magnesium in the 'citrate' form, which is the best for absorption, vitamin D and boron. Ideal for women at risk of osteoporosis.

READ THE LABELS

Some products do not supply very much of the minerals you need. Do look carefully, and ask the manager or pharmacist for help if you aren't sure. One well-known brand, for example, costs around £4 for 25 days' worth and supplies only 360 mg of the 1250 mg of calcium you would need if you were breast feeding.

Problems of muscles and joints

Muscle and joint problems are universal. Virtually no human being escapes some disorder of these structures during their lifetime. Both in my practice as an osteopath and in the phone-in programmes, a large proportion of the inquiries which I deal with revolve around these structures.

Joint disease is nothing new – even ancient skeletons recovered by archaeologists show signs of arthritic disease. Man was not designed to stand on two feet and the consequent stresses and strains imposed on the joints of the spine, hips, knees and ankles all add to the increasing prevalence of arthritic disease and to the ubiquitous problem of back ache. Add to this our modern civilised lifestyle which is far more sedentary and less active than that of our forebears, the dramatic changes in our diet during the last hundred years, and the increasing prevalence of obesity, and we have a good witches' brew of aggravating factors. Furthermore, the stresses of life in our 20th-century world all combine to produce situations which encourage the build-up of muscular tension. As this tension becomes more chronic it leads to the development of fibrositis, postural faults, tension headaches and a multitude of other stress-related disorders.

Arthritis

The word 'arthritis' means simply inflammation of a joint. There are a number of different diseases which produce arthritis, all of which have the same common factor. That is to say, they involve lesions of the connective tissue. These connective tissue diseases are divided broadly into two main categories: (A) The diseases in which symptoms are caused by inflammatory changes, for example, rheumatoid arthritis, ankylosing spondylitis, systemic lupus erythematosus (SLE) and gout. Also in this group are the various forms of osteo-chondritis. (B) Diseases in which the symptoms are caused through degenerative changes in the connective tissue such as osteo-arthrosis, inter-vertebral disc problems and spondylosis.

Rheumatoid arthritis

This disease affects many joints, mainly in the extremities. The specific causes of this disease are still somewhat obscure, but it is an illness which runs a prolonged course of many years, often starting with general muscular pain and stiffness, tiredness, tingling in the hands and feet, and then producing swellings of the joints of the fingers and toes. The progress of rheumatoid arthritis is often a series of ups and downs, acute phases in which the patient feels extremely unwell, followed by periods of remission of varying lengths.

The disease usually begins at around the age of 40. It affects women three times as frequently as men and it is not uncommon for there to be a family history of rheumatoid arthritis. There may be a connection with disturbance of the immune responses and there is nearly always the development of the rheumatoid factor. The disease is sometimes triggered, and during its course frequently aggravated, by severe emotional disturbances and excessive anxiety and overwork.

During acute phases of the illness, joints are frequently immobilised and the patient advised to take complete rest. Drug therapy relies on the use of the anti-inflammatory and pain-killing drugs, so that aspirin and a range of newer anti-inflammatories are used, though these are not without side effects. Cortico-steroids do have a powerful anti-inflammatory action but the dangers of long-term treatment with these drugs must always be borne in mind. Intramuscular injections of gold salts are used but can also produce serious side effects. Where there has been severe joint damage, surgery is a means of relieving the patient's discomfort. Replacement of joints, especially hip joint replacement, which is very successful, fusion of joints to prevent movement and removal of some joints may be done in extreme cases.

Ankylosing spondylitis

This is a gradually progressive inflammatory arthritis of the joints of the spine. It most commonly affects males between the ages of 20 and 40. In fact, men suffer from this problem ten times more frequently than women. It develops slowly and any young man who has a history of frequent attacks of back ache for no very obvious reason should be regarded with some suspicion. X-rays of the lower part of the spine and the sacroiliac joints are vital since it is in these joints that the first typical changes occur (bamboo spine). In time the entire spine becomes progressively more rigid and the joints between the ribs and the spine are also affected. This can produce severe breathing problems as it limits the expansion of the chest wall. Postural deformities are also common and, in severe cases, the patient can become badly incapacitated.

Systemic lupus erythematosus (SLE)

This disease also involves the connective tissue in many parts of the body and again it is believed to be due to some changes in the body's own immune responses. Young women are most frequently affected, ten times more than men and, during the child-bearing years, fifteen times more commonly than men. SLE has been known to be triggered by a number of factors, unaccustomed exposure to sunlight, infection, emotional stress and some drugs, particularly penicillin, sulphonamides, anti-convulsants and, occasionally, oral contraceptives.

The illness is typified by fever with acute joint pain which moves from joint to joint throughout the body. There are often skin eruptions on the face and hands, the patients are tired, anorexic and anaemic. There is frequently a 'butterfly' rash on the face.

Orthodox treatment involves the use of steroids in the most acute cases, although the anti-malarial drug, chloroquine, has produced good results in the less acute patients.

Gout

Gout is not the music hall joke illness of crusty colonels drinking large quantities of port. An acute attack of gout can be excruciatingly painful. It usually affects the big toe joint but can spread to other joints as the disease progresses. Since gout is caused by an inborn fault in the body's ability to metabolise purine, it follows that gout is largely a hereditary disorder. In fact, well over half the people who suffer from gout will have a family history of the disease. It seldom appears before the age of 40 and is very rare in women. It is no longer thought that gout is due to an excessive intake of foods with high purine content but there is evidence to suggest that attacks can be triggered off by dietary indiscretions in patients predisposed to the disease. An acute attack can also be caused by injury, excessive exercise and sometimes as a result of surgery.

In the early stages of the disease the acute attacks are infrequent, with long periods of relief in between. However, as time goes on, the attacks occur more frequently and last longer. Finally, there is consistent pain, loss of movement and deformity of the joint. The disease spreads to other joints, particularly in the ankles, wrists and hands, followed by knees, shoulders, hips and elbows. Chalky deposits of urates called tophi then begin to appear around the joints affected and in the cartilage of the ears.

The commonest medical form of treatment for gout is the use of non-steroidal anti-inflammatory drugs during the acute episodes, followed by long-term therapy with Allopurinol. Due to the effectiveness of the drugs, patients are seldom advised to make any dietary changes.

Osteo-arthritis (O/A)

This is a degenerative disease of the weight-bearing surfaces of the joints. The disease affects both the cartilage and the surface of the bone, with the cartilage wearing away and additional irregular new bone growing around the edges of the affected joints.

O/A can affect both spinal and peripheral joints. It is *not*, as so often stated, just a degenerative disease of old age, but it can result from many different causes, particularly changes in metabolism, inflammation or direct mechanical injury to the joint's surfaces. Hobbies, sports and occupations can all have a direct bearing on the development of osteo-arthritis. For instance, arthritis of the spine is common amongst the heavy industrial occupations, coal-mining, the building industry, dockers, agricultural workers, whereas arthritis of the extremities can be caused by repetitive movements, for example, ticket collector's thumb.

Heavy manual labour can also produce arthritis of the hips, knees and ankles. O/A is also likely to occur in any joint which has been damaged by traumatic injury. Misalignment of fractures can also cause O/A in adjacent joints.

The most common symptoms of all forms of osteo-arthritis are pain, immobility and stiffness, often accompanied by the creaking and cracking noises of crepitus. Periods of inactivity or overactivity can both exacerbate the condition. O/A of the spine most frequently occurs in the neck and lumbar regions, although it is found in other parts of the back.

Whilst the degenerative changes that occur in the bone and cartilage due to osteo-arthritis are not reversible, much can be done to alleviate the symptoms and to slow down the progression of the disease.

The most usual medical treatments are the use of the non-steroidal anti-inflammatory drugs and also the injection of steroids into affected joints. Surgery is also used with great effect in the replacement of arthritic hip joints, an operation which has brought enormous relief to countless thousands of people. Surgery for the replacement of knee joints is not so successful and many orthopaedic surgeons have abandoned this procedure.

Surgery can also be used to fix arthritic joints and to remove debris from within the joint space.

Sensible approaches to the treatment of joint disorders

All sufferers from joint disease, whether inflammatory connective tissue disease or degenerative arthritic disease, have the ability to help themselves considerably. The simple expedient of changing eating habits can bring relief in varying degrees in all these conditions.

Rheumatoid arthritis, ankylosing spondylitis, SLE – in all these illnesses it is advisable to remove from the daily diet all red meats, meat products, red wines, port, sherry, madeira, refined carbohydrates, sugar, coffee, strong tea and *all* dairy products. Increase the quantities of fish, poultry, green vegetables, salads, fruits, nuts, whole grain cereals and vegetable proteins. Herbal teas and fruit juices (not citrus) are an excellent alternative to normal tea.

Those suffering from osteo-arthritis should follow the same rules but they may include reasonable quantities of dairy products in their diet.

Every surplus pound of body weight increases the strain on the weight-bearing joints. Therefore it is vital to reduce weight to the minimum optimum level.

The maintenance of mobility and muscle tone is another key factor in overcoming all the arthritic problems. Regular exercise of a non-weight-bearing variety such as swimming, the use of a stationary bicycle, hydrotherapy or any other form of non-weight-bearing gentle movement will all help to maintain muscle tone and flexibility.

Manipulative treatment

Osteopathy and chiropractic have a great deal to offer to the arthritis sufferer. The maintenance of good posture and the restoration of maximum possible movement to affected joints are all of benefit, both in the relief of pain and discomfort and in the long-term course of the illness. Manipulation, however, is specifically contra-indicated in the acute inflammatory processes such as rheumatoid arthritis, SLE and ankylosing spondylitis.

Herbal remedies

Most of the modern anti-inflammatory drugs are derived from the original basis of aspirin, but the side effects of these drugs are well known. Aspirin, whose chemical name is salicylic acid, was originally derived from the willow tree whose name is salix. There are modern herbal extracts available, the most effective of which I have found is Bio-Strath Willow formula, which is a mixture of extract of willow and primula. It has a powerful anti-inflammatory effect but does not have any of the disturbing side effects of the synthetic drugs. This can be taken long-term with no dangers whatsoever. In addition, celery seed tablets are useful for their alkaline properties, and parsley tea can also be beneficial as it stimulates the body's elimination of fluids. Put a heaped teaspoon-ful of finely chopped parsley into a cup of boiling water, cover and leave till cool. Strain the tea and sip occasionally throughout the day, consuming the entire cup over a 24-hour period.

Massaging painful areas gently with a massage oil containing rosemary and lavender will help to relieve local pain.

Naturopathy

Whilst heat may seem to relieve discomfort and swelling, cold compresses are more effective in stimulating the circulation and relieving inflammation. A large bag of frozen peas makes an excellent ice pack. The affected area should be covered with a thin cotton cloth (a larger handkerchief or thin cotton teatowel is ideal), the bag of peas applied to the affected area and left for eight minutes. Remove the bag of peas and give the area a very gentle rub with a warm flannel and then dry with a towel. Repeat this ice pack treatment twice daily, as necessary. Mark the packet of peas with a large, easily identifiable mark and return it to the freezer. Since you are going to be using these regularly they should not be eaten as they will have been partially thawed and refrozen repeatedly.

Muscular aches and pains can be relieved by soaking in a hot epsom salts bath for about twenty minutes each evening. Three tablespoons of epsom salts should be dissolved in the water and thoroughly mixed. For severe arthritic inflammation, a bath containing Kneipp juniper oil is extremely effective. The bath should be comfortably hot and you should soak in it for at least fifteen to twenty minutes on alternate nights.

Taking some additional vitamins and minerals can also help in both rheumatoid and osteo-arthritis. A dose of 200 mg of calcium pantothenate, 100 mg of nicotinamide and 500 mg of vitamin C taken daily will be of benefit.

Acupuncture

Self-help with acupressure is beneficial in the relief of the acute symptoms of all arthritic conditions. See relevant diagrams.

Whilst all the above will help you to help yourself, the arthritic conditions respond extremely well to professional complementary therapy. The best forms of treatment are a combination of osteopathy, naturopathy and acupuncture.

Bunions (Hallux vulgus)

A bunion is a large inflamed swelling on the outside of the joint between the big toe and the foot. Bunions frequently run in families where there is a tendency for the big toe to turn inwards towards the other toes, but they are nearly always totally avoidable.

Bunions are most frequently caused by ill-fitting high fashion shoes and consequently are more common in women than men. Some years ago the fashion for 'winkle picker' shoes in men triggered off a virtual epidemic of this painful and disabling condition in the male population too.

What happens to your child's feet now decides whether or not they get bunions later. Here are some simple rules:

(1) Be very careful with socks: make sure that you buy the right size for your child and remember that feet grow and socks shrink.

(2) Be careful with all-in-one clothes for babies. The ubiquitous babygrow can restrict the child's foot and cause compression of the toes. Cut off the babygrow's feet if it is tight.

(3) Do not buy one-size socks because for every force there is an equal and opposite force and the stretch sock will compress the foot.

(4) Do not put shoes on your baby until he or she is walking and then make sure that there is ample room for the feet to spread within the shoe.

(5) Be very careful where you buy your children's shoes. If you walk into the shop and the assistant asks you what size shoe the child takes, that's the time to walk out again. No child should be fitted with shoes until the foot has been properly measured for length and width.

(6) Do not let your children, especially your daughters, persuade you into buying them high-heeled pointed shoes as these will inevitably lead to deformities. There is nothing wrong in a pair of fashionable party shoes if these are only worn occasionally, but for everyday use the right fit is essential.

(7) A useful tip is to take a tin of talcum powder when you go shoe shopping. Sprinkle a little powder into the shoe, get your child to try it on, take the shoe off and look inside. You will see that the talcum powder forms a very neat outline of the toes and you can see just how much room there is inside the shoe.

(8) The question of trainers is one which arouses all sorts of misgivings in parents. The properly designed, well-made trainer is in fact suitable footwear for children. They are usually well constructed and round-toed, leaving ample room for adequate movement and growth of the foot, and since the material is usually soft they do not restrict the shape of the foot.

If you already have bunions see Arthritis (page 83) for general instructions on diet and other forms of self-help. In addition there are a number of exercises which you will find beneficial. Rolling the feet backward and forward on a bottle or a large rolling pin, or picking up pencils under your toes and heel-to-toe walking in bare feet, will all help. Every time you sit in the bath you should give your toes a really good massage and wiggle them about under the hot water. Using a large rubber band looped over both big toes, then sitting with legs outstretched and heels together, you should rotate the legs outwards forming a 'V' between the two feet and pulling the big toes towards each other. Repeat this twenty or thirty times at least twice a day. The use of small foam rubber toe spacers between the big toe and the second toe is also a great help. Contrast bathing of the feet is also useful. You should have a bucket filled with hot water containing a tablespoonful of epsom salts and a bucket full of cold water. Place the feet in the hot water for one minute and in the cold water for fifteen seconds. Repeat ten times each evening.

Osteopathic manipulation, whilst not being a cure for the already deformed joint, will improve the mobility and prevent the joint from deteriorating even further. Hopefully with this sort of treatment you will be able to avoid the use of surgery, since this treatment for bunions is not always totally satisfactory.

Back pain

Back pain of one sort or another is certainly the most common single problem from which the British public suffers. Back ache costs British industry more than £1000 million a year in lost productivity and something like half the population of this country have had back pain at some time or another. Back pain can strike anyone at any time and once you have had an acute episode of back ache, there is a one in two chance that you will get a recurrence.

Whilst osteopaths deal with many muscular and skeletal problems, as well as other diseases too, it is in the treatment of back pain that they come into their own. Well over half the patients seen by myself and my colleagues arrive in our consulting rooms with some form of back problem, and they all have one thing in common – they are beset by old wives' tales. So let's dispel some of the myths about the back.

'Slipped disc' – there's no such thing as a slipped disc. A disc can rupture or bulge or become worn and narrow but it cannot slip.

'Back ache means there is something wrong with my spine' – not necessarily. There are many causes of back ache, some of them quite trivial.

'I've had back ache for months. Isn't an operation the only thing that will make me better?' – no is the simple answer. Surgery is the last resort, most people get better without it.

'I suppose I shall have to give up my job' – unless you are a docker, a coalman, a miner, or something of the sort, the answer is usually no.

'The doctor says he can't find anything wrong with my back and has prescribed valium. Is the pain all in my mind?' – if there is pain then it's real. Sometimes psychological stresses can be an important aggravating factor.

'I've been told to give up all sport in case I injure my back even more' – you must not give up sport altogether. Hurt is not the same as harm. You may, however, have to change to a different type of sporting activity.

There are a variety of causes of back pain. Pain can be triggered by a damaged or worn disc bulging under pressure, and this in turn presses against the ligaments of the spine which are very sensitive to pain. Nerve root pressure can be caused by a ruptured disc. In this situation the wall of the disc breaks and the jelly in the centre squeezes out causing direct pressure on the spinal nerves. This type of pain is very acute and frightening. It is also extremely disabling. Pressure on the nerve roots can also cause referred pain, particularly down the leg, which is sciatica (see Slipped disc, page 100). Inflammation of the joints is a frequent cause of back pain and this can be the result of injury or of an inflammatory condition like arthritis. Muscle spasm is probably the commonest cause of mild back ache. This can be the result of occupational stresses, poor posture, bad seating, injury or strain of the muscles. Any of these can cause the muscles to contract and go into spasm, and, if there is an underlying problem with the disc, the increase in pressure exerted by the muscles can aggravate the pain caused by the disc as well.

Other diseases may also produce back pain: digestive problems, gall stones, kidney disease, gynaecological disorders, tumours and even some types of cancer. So you can see how important it is that you consult a properly trained and qualified osteopath, since the diagnosis of the exact cause of the back pain is essential before any form of treatment is undertaken.

Treatment and prevention of back pain

In all episodes of back pain speed is of the essence. It is imperative that you consult your osteopath as soon as possible, since once a pattern of muscle spasm has set in, it is far more difficult to relieve this and so get to the underlying cause of the problem. I would far rather see twenty patients with back ache to whom I say, 'Go home, have a hot bath, it will be better in the morning', than miss out on one patient who suffers for months on end with niggling back ache before seeking advice merely because he didn't like to bother anybody. Once this happens you are much more likely to be involved in lengthy and costly courses of treatment.

When I first started in practice in 1964 most patients came to the osteopath as a last resort. They had already paraded their back through the GP's surgery, the physiotherapy department, the hospital consultant's room, and had run the whole gamut of orthodox treatment – bed rest, corsets, drugs, traction, physiotherapy, injections, and finally when threatened with surgery, they decided to do something more to help themselves, and seek the advice of an osteopath. Happily, today more and more people come initially to the osteopath and say, 'Please can you help or do I need to see the doctor?'

It is in the area of back treatment that the manipulative therapists, both osteopaths and chiropractors, come into their own. The main approach is that of the holistic therapist. The osteopath starts to make his diagnosis the instant he sees the patient either getting out of his car or walking in the door of the consulting room. How does he walk, how does he move, how does he sit and stand, does he have any obvious postural faults, what is the level of pain and discomfort that the patient is suffering? A detailed case history must be taken, a full physical examination given, and the patient must take his clothes off, for how can you diagnose a back problem without looking at the back? How often I have heard the tale of patients who had been backwards and forwards to their GP for months on end with back ache and the GP had never once asked the patient to take off his shirt.

Once the osteopath has completed his examination, he is likely to begin some form of treatment straight away, and, depending upon the severity of the patient's condition and the degree of pain which they are suffering, he may either choose to do purely soft tissue and massage treatment, or to administer some form of manipulative therapy.

There will be situations where the osteopath's diagnosis will reveal that the patient is one of the unfortunate few (probably around 0.1 per cent of back sufferers) who may need surgery to resolve their problems, and in this situation he will almost certainly refer the patient to an orthopaedic surgeon.

A vital component of osteopathic treatment is to encourage patients to help themselves with the problem and to this end the osteopath will certainly prescribe a gradually progressive series of exercises to improve the current situation and to strengthen and improve the mobility of the spine in order to prevent recurrent episodes. Sadly, most patients very soon forget how painful their back was and give up doing the exercises. This is a great mistake, since, particularly with backs, prevention is better than cure.

There are a number of things which you can and should do to help yourself.

Do not allow yourself to become or remain overweight as this increases the strain on all your spinal joints. Ensure that you keep active. Do the exercises which you have been prescribed and take up some form of non-weight-bearing exercise – swimming is ideal.

Make sure that your bed is firm and supports you adequately. Be particularly careful how you use your back, learn to bend your knees when lifting, do not carry excessively heavy weights; when doing jobs around the house or the garden try to have two or three different jobs on the go at the same time so that you spend fifteen minutes at each one, thus avoiding prolonged periods in fixed positions.

At work, insist that you have a proper chair at your desk, that it's adjustable, that the back will support you in the right position. If you're a secretary you need a footstool. If you're a draughtsman, architect, artist or machine operator – try to ensure that your work-surface is at the right height for your back. If necessary, stand on boards or raise or lower the height of your working surface. Do not slump around in an armchair watching the telly in the evening, and especially don't fall asleep in the armchair. If you're tired, go to bed. If you want to watch the television make sure you are sitting in a well-supported upright chair with a high back which also supports your head. Don't allow yourself to be conned into buying very expensive orthopaedic beds or chairs. They are no better than those made by the reputable furniture and bed manufacturers which are normally considerably cheaper.

Car seats are a common source of problems, especially to people who drive for a living. Most of them are poorly designed and do not provide adequate lumbar support except in the most expensive of cars. If you are a professional driver with a chronic back problem it's worth considering having a special car seat fitted. There are several on the market, particularly those made by Putnams, who also make inexpensive support cushions which can be placed in the back of the seat. You will find the address at the back of the book.

There are no miracle cures for back problems. The only sensible approach is the long-term care of your back coupled with the correct form of treatment, which is nearly always manipulative therapy.

Acupuncture can help to relieve the acute pain of back ache, although it will not resolve mechanical disturbances of the spine. There are acupressure points which you can use yourself to relieve immediate discomfort (see diagram on page 94).

For back pain which is basically caused by muscular stresses remedial massage is extremely beneficial but is only effective as a palliative unless the underlying causes of muscular tension can be eliminated. The use of alternate hot and cold compresses or cold packs will also help to relieve the acute pain of most forms of back ache. Finally it is worth considering the role of psychology in the treatment of back disorders. Whilst it is seldom true that underlying psychological problems are the sole cause of back ache, they do frequently become a major factor, especially when one is dealing with chronic back sufferers. After all, any form of chronic pain is

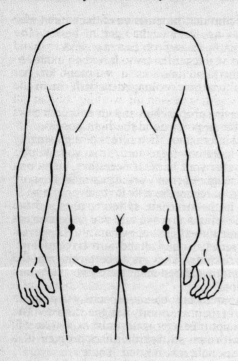

Acupressure points for the relief of back ache. The points (shown by dots) should be treated with continuous firm pressure and massaged in small circles for one to three minutes, as necessary, repeated four to five times daily, or more frequently for the relief of severe pain. Use a finger or a small rounded implement such as the cap of a ballpoint pen

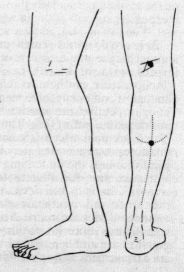

depressing. One must also consider the situation of the patient who has a vested interest in staying ill rather than getting better. The high-powered executive with business problems may wish to avoid going back to his office; the young mother who is finding it hard to cope with new babies may see this as a way out of her responsibilities; the agricultural worker may view with alarm the onset of winter and yet another season of working out in all weathers. All these are mostly subconscious and unrealised factors which can be elicited with the help of a good psychotherapist.

The concept of the back sufferer as a malingerer merely swinging the lead to avoid work is greatly exaggerated. In a quarter of a century of practice I don't suppose I've seen more than a dozen of this type of patient. To the experienced practitioner there is no mistaking the patient who is in pain with an acute back problem.

To all those thousands of you who are suffering or who have endured back problems, I would urge you to see a competent osteopath or chiropractor at the earliest opportunity. His special diagnostic skills, together with the use of all the normal technological developments – X-rays, blood tests, scans if necessary – and the growing co-operation between manipulative therapists, GPs and orthopaedic surgeons, will give you the best possible chance of a speedy recovery from your acute condition and even more importantly a brighter long-term outlook for the future. The manipulative therapist will not take over your problem, but he will encourage you to work with him so that the ultimate goal of a normal existence free of back pain may become reality.

Cramp

This is a sudden but acutely painful contraction of muscles which occurs frequently in the calves but is also possible in any of the muscles of the neck, back, face or abdomen. Cramp is often related to occupation, and writers, typists, pianists, drummers, violinists and, most commonly, athletes, are prone to it. These are all people using repetitive movements of the same muscle groups over prolonged periods of time. The spasm of muscles is normally caused by an accumulation of lactic acid in the muscle tissue which promotes contraction of the muscle fibres and the ensuing violent painful cramp.

It's common for athletes to take salt to prevent or alleviate cramp. This is a bad idea, since only the most extreme heat exhaustion and resultant loss of salt will respond to this particular treatment. Modern nutritional thinking suggests that additional potassium is more satisfactory. Kelp tablets, calcium lactate and quinine have also been useful in treating recurrent cramp. Bananas are a convenient source of potassium.

The sudden onset of cramp in any muscle can sometimes be alleviated quickly by stretching the muscle against the contraction.

Osteopathic treatment is useful, although it is likely to involve deep massage rather than manipulation, unless there is a spinal problem causing pressure on the nerve roots which supply the muscles of the affected area, in which case manipulation is indicated.

The homoeopathic remedies nux vomica and arnica are both helpful.

Naturopathic treatment with contrast bathing, hot and cold water to the legs if those are affected, and mustard footbaths three times weekly will help. To make a footbath use one tablespoon of mustard power and enough water to cover the feet and ankles. Immerse the feet in the water for five minutes, splashing the calves liberally and dry briskly with a rough towel to stimulate the circulation.

Recurrent cramp responds well to a daily dose of 1000 mg of dolomite, 400 iu of vitamin E daily and 500 mg of potassium.

Where cramp is the result of emotional stress being transferred into muscular contraction, as is commonly the cause in writer's cramp and musician's cramp, then the use of relaxation techniques to help combat the stress problem is essential if a long-term cure is to be effected.

Fibrositis

Fibrositis literally means inflammation of muscle fibres. This is a very common problem all too frequently ignored by doctors or, even worse, dismissed as an inevitable consequence of growing old. Small nodules of fibrous tissue arise deep within the large muscles of the body. These, rather like the sand in an oyster, irritate the surrounding tissues which then too become fibrous. The fibrous nodules grow and eventually can cause chronic and severe pain or discomfort. Most commonly, fibrositis occurs in the large muscles of the back, the muscles of the neck and shoulders and also in the muscles of the buttocks.

This condition can arise as a result of poor posture, or previous injury which affects the way in which the body is used, following severe stress to the muscles such as heavy lifting, unaccustomed painting or decorating, or a sudden bout of enthusiastic gardening. Fibrositis can also arise after prolonged periods of sitting, especially when concentrating on operating machines like computer terminals, telex and fax machines, calculators and typewriters.

Stress, tension and anxiety all too frequently result in tension of the muscles, especially those of the back and shoulders, with resulting fibrositis.

Any osteopath or masseur, practitioners who constantly have

their hands on patients' bodies, can normally pinpoint areas of fibrositis purely through their well-developed sense of touch.

Osteopathic treatment is important in the relief of this condition. It is essential to determine the underlying causes and to treat them accordingly in addition to local deep neuro-muscular techniques of massage to the fibrous areas. It is important to avoid obesity and to maintain some form of regular exercise appropriate to the age and physical condition of the patient. Hot epsom salt baths, the application of a heat lamp or a well-covered hot water bottle will all help to reduce the discomfort, as will the use of herbal anti-inflammatory preparations like Bio-Strath willow formula. However, all palliative measures will only be temporary unless the correct manipulative treatment is applied to remove the underlying cause of the condition.

Naturopathic treatment with a diet low in 'acid-forming' foods (e.g. meat, sugar, eggs) and increasing the quantities of raw vegetables, whole grains and fresh fruit, but excluding citrus fruits, should be encouraged. Contrast bathing with alternate hot and cold cloths always finishing with cold, and ending up with a friction rub using a rough towel, will also help.

Relaxation therapy should also be encouraged as this will be a big step towards controlling the underlying tensions which create fibrositis.

A high dose of calcium pantothenate – 2000 mg daily – should be taken until the pain subsides, and thereafter a daily dose of thiamine (vitamin B1) of 50 mg should be continued for up to six weeks.

Frozen shoulder

This common complaint often results in sheer desperation for the many people who suffer from it. The shoulder joint is extremely complex and has a large range of movements. Because of this it is more likely to be affected by pain and restriction of movement than many of the other joints.

This appallingly painful condition can appear for no apparent reason. The pain is so severe as to make some movements virtually impossible. Simple activities like doing up a bra, combing the hair, or getting a wallet from your hip pocket become agonisingly difficult. Because movements of the shoulder joint produce such pain, sufferers tend to use the whole shoulder girdle to lift the arm and hand. This naturally limits the mobility of the joint and encourages the formation of fibrositis and adhesions. These in turn make movement even more difficult and so we end up with a self-perpetuating vicious circle.

The administration of heat, physiotherapy, anti-inflammatory drugs and steroid injections can all provide temporary relief

Problems of muscles and joints

sometimes, but patients with this condition are often told that they can expect their symptoms to persist for anything up to two years and, after this length of time, it is unlikely that full normal movement will return to the joint.

Osteopathic treatment for frozen shoulder is certainly the treatment of choice, particularly where this can be combined with acupuncture which will help to relieve the acute pain. Massage, contrast bathing and manipulation of the shoulder joint and the joints of the neck form an important part of the treatment. Ice packs, preferably using a large bag of frozen peas moulded to the shape of the shoulder, are of great benefit since this stimulates the circulation to the deeper tissues and encourages faster healing of the damaged areas. Exercises are vital and a regime of progressively more complex movements will maintain and improve the mobility and also prevent muscle wastage during the course of treatment.

Herbal remedies and vitamin therapy are the same as for fibrositis.

Occasionally the symptoms of frozen shoulder are produced by the deposit of calcium in the deep tendons of the shoulder joint. Where this is the case manipulation is not likely to achieve any benefits, although massage, exercise and all the other self-help treatments are very important in maintaining the overall health of the joint. In this situation, surgery to remove the calcium deposits is sometimes the only answer.

Headache caused by tension

Headaches may be a symptom of some other underlying disease or they may commonly be the result of postural problems and physical stress and tension. See also Blood pressure (page 124), Whiplash (page 106), Sinusitis (page 115), Menstrual disorders (page 154) and Migraine (page 190).

By far the most common cause of headaches is tension in the large muscles at the back of the neck and shoulder, combined with problems affecting the spinal joints in the neck and shoulder region.

Eye problems can also be a cause of headaches and if your head aches consistently after activities involving a lot of reading or long periods looking at the VDU on a computer terminal, then the first step is to have your eyes tested. More commonly these occupational headaches are the result of poor posture in your work situation and you should look at ways of improving this by adjusting chairs, benches, desks or even the simple expedient of moving your telephone to a more convenient position. I remember one particular patient, a left-handed young lady, who had suffered continual pains in the neck and shoulders and headaches for three years since moving to a new job. I could find no medical reasons for

98

these headaches and all the normal tests were negative. She worked as a receptionist in a busy film studio, so I asked her to sit at my desk and rearrange the objects on it in the same way they were in her office. The first thing she did was to place the telephone on the right-hand side of the desk. For three years, every time the phone rang, she had been reaching across the desk with her left hand to pick up the telephone, hold it to her left ear, whilst having to bend to the right because the lead on the telephone was too short. The simple expedient of moving the telephone to the left side of the desk resolved her problem in a matter of weeks, not however without a little help from osteopathic treatment.

Swallowing aspirins is not the answer for dealing with recurrent headaches. Firstly, they are likely to cause severe gastric disturbance in the long term, and secondly this is not getting to the root of the problem. I see many patients who get up in the morning and take two aspirins in case they get a headache. These people are addicted to the use of aspirins. You must endeavour to find out why you are getting headaches caused by stress and tension. It is obvious to say that you need to deal with these underlying problems if you are to achieve long-term relief from this depressing and debilitating condition.

Osteopathic treatment will help you, with correction of postural faults, massage and exercises to relieve fibrositis, tense muscles and

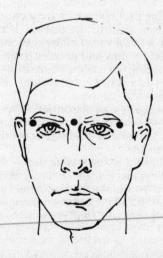

Acupressure points for the relief of headache. For
acupressure instructions, see caption on page 94

improve mobility and above all the appropriate advice regarding the way in which you use your body. Acupuncture can also be a considerable aid to the relief of headaches and there are some useful pressure points which you can use for yourself. See diagram.

The Alexander Technique of postural re-education is often important for the long-term prevention of recurrent headaches, since learning this technique re-establishes the correct relationship between your head, neck and trunk and thereby eliminates unnecessary and wasteful muscle activity.

Herbal treatment with 'antispasmodic' tincture containing skull-cap and valerian is useful. A teaspoon of the tincture in a cup of warm water sweetened with two teaspoons of honey will give rapid relief and you can massage the undiluted tincture over the forehead, temples and base of the neck. Homoeopathic treatment with arnica or belladonna can also be used. Vitamin B complex in a high potency dose taken daily is also advisable.

Restless legs (See also Cramp)

This condition, which is commoner in women than in men, is seldom properly diagnosed. Strictly speaking it is a condition arising from blood disorders and doesn't truly belong in this section of the book. However, it is so frequently confused with muscular cramp that I include it here because this is where most people will look for it.

This is a disturbing problem which frequently disrupts the social life, travelling or even visits to the cinema. It interrupts sleep and can be a major factor in the onset of depression.

It is characterised by pins and needles, pain in the legs, jerking movements and burning sensations when sitting. The only way that the patient can get any relief is by walking. But on sitting down again the symptoms soon reappear.

This problem is an early sign of iron deficiency and it can be one of the first symptoms of anaemia. Heavy periods, piles, diverticulitis, or any condition which causes gradual but continuous loss of blood can be a causative factor.

It is helpful to have a naturopathic diet rich in iron-containing foods (eggs, wholegrain cereals, liver, green leafy vegetables) taken together with a natural iron supplement containing folic acid and 200 iu of vitamin E daily. Contrast bathing of the legs in hot and cold water (finishing with cold) will provide temporary relief during an acute episode.

Slipped disc (Prolapsed intervertebral disc)

There is in fact no such thing as a slipped disc. The disc acts as a shock absorber between each pair of vertebrae in the spine and since these discs are subjected to continuous stresses and strains and wear and tear, various things can happen to them. They can wear thin, they can rupture, they can bulge or they can be affected by some disease processes, but they cannot slip.

The purpose of the intervertebral disc is to maintain the correct amount of separation between the individual vertebrae and thus enable the spine to function in its proper manner. The discs are made up of a thick outer membrane rather like a plastic bag containing a nucleus of thick jelly. When pressure is applied to the discs they tend to shrink because the fluids inside the disc are squeezed out. At rest the discs absorb body fluids and swell again, pushing the vertebrae apart, and this is the main reason for bed rest being the first and most effective treatment of acute disc injuries.

A disc can be damaged by abnormal stresses on a normal disc, normal stresses on a normal disc when the body is unprepared, or by normal stresses on an abnormal disc. Rupture of the wall of the disc enables the central jelly to squeeze out through the damaged area and to press against the nerve roots coming from the spinal canal. It is this mechanism that causes the acute crippling pain of the so-called 'slipped disc'. It is quite impossible to correct this type of injury by manipulation and practitioners claiming to 'push your disc back into place' are talking nonsense. Imagine trying to get the toothpaste back into the tube – it's the same problem.

However, many nerve root problems are caused not by ruptures of the disc but by a general bulging of the disc to one side or other of the vertebral column. In this situation manipulative treatment can relieve the uneven pressures on the disc surface and allow the disc to return to its normal shape and in this way resolve the symptoms.

Long-term stresses such as obesity, heavy manual work, or very strenuous sporting activities, or even pregnancy, can gradually weaken the wall of the disc so much that the final straw which breaks the camel's back is sometimes a very minor incident. Most patients who end up on my couch with an acute disc problem have done it by some small movement – tying a shoelace, bending to pick up a pencil, or simply getting out of the car in an awkward way. Very few of them arrive as the result of one single traumatic injury.

The immediate result of a prolapsed disc is acute violent pain. It is caused by direct pressure on the nerve root and the resulting protective muscle spasm that follows. There may also be pain, numbness and/or pins and needles radiating through the buttocks, down the leg, right into the foot and toes (sciatica). In extreme cases muscle weakness and, after some weeks, muscle wastage can be apparent. Any difficulty in passing urine is cause for concern and medical advice should be sought immediately.

101

The sooner that treatment can be done, the quicker the patient will benefit. The first step is to encourage complete and total rest, either on a very firm bed or on a thin mattress on the floor. When the pain is severe, manipulative treatment may not be possible, but the use of massage and gentle mobilisation, alternate hot and cold packs to the lower part of the spine and ultrasound therapy will also help to relax the large muscles of the back which will be in spasm.

As mobility returns, so manipulative treatment can begin. This will be aimed at improving the mobility of the spinal joints, relieving pressure on the affected disc and its associated nerve roots, and gradual rehabilitation back to normal function.

Large doses of calcium pantothenate, up to 2000 mg daily for the first few days, and then gradually reducing the dose to 50 mg daily, will help as an anti-inflammatory, especially if used concurrently with Bio-Strath willow and primula formula.

Acupuncture is an effective way of relieving the acute pain of disc problems, although of course it cannot realign mechanical faults in the spine itself. Use the pressure points in the diagram for self-help during the acute phase.

Defend your discs

As with all back problems, prevention is better than cure. Learning how to lift and carry, sit and stand, work and play in the most effective way to protect your back is essential. Bending forwards exerts the greatest amount of pressure on the intervertebral discs and this is true whether you are sitting or standing. Never forget that if you are carrying heavy weights, carry them as close to your body as possible. Any weight held at arm's length exerts fifteen times more than its own weight in pressure on the discs at the lower part of your back.

Above all, keep your spine healthy by maintaining correct body weight and taking part in some form of regular physical activity. It doesn't matter whether you are 8 or 80, there is no need to avoid physical exertion as long as you tailor your activities to your own particular abilities.

Not all disc problems can be satisfactorily resolved through the use of complementary techniques. A small percentage of patients will need surgery and the competent manipulator will know when this time comes. Thankfully the old animosities between orthopaedic surgeons and osteopaths are dying away and most highly trained professionals work happily together.

If surgery does turn out to be the only solution in your case, do make sure that you get yourself in as healthy a state as possible, by eating well, by taking extra vitamins, by preparing yourself for your time in hospital, and, as soon as you are sufficiently recovered, go

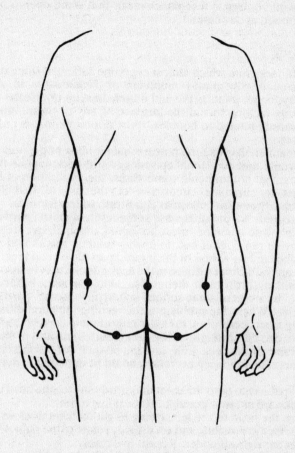

**Acupressure points for the relief of acute pain arising
from disc problems. For acupressure instructions, see
caption on page 94**

back to your osteopath as he will be the ideal person to make sure that you maintain your spine in a fit, proper and healthy manner. Today's microsurgical techniques mean that some operations can be performed as day cases.

Stiff neck

The stiff neck from which almost everyone suffers at some time or another is nearly always muscular or ligamentous in origin. Naturally, bone, joint, nerve and muscle injuries or disease can be underlying factors, but in the absence of any of these, muscular strain, mostly related to hobbies, sport or occupation, is probably the reason.

The maintenance of good posture and mobility of the neck joints is important, and occasional episodes of stiff neck may be treated with massage, hot and cold compresses, the application of herbal liniments to stimulate circulation or the use of herbal anti-inflammatory medicines such as Bio-Strath willow formula.

Where there is a physical cause as the result of injury, particularly the whiplash so common in car accidents, manipulative treatment will provide rapid relief but, following trauma, this should not be undertaken unless X-rays of the injured part have been seen.

Repeated attacks of stiffness in the neck muscles may be associated with fibrositis, arthritis or rheumatism, while an acute onset of stiff neck can be a sign of some serious underlying disease, particularly meningitis. Where the problem is the result of postural difficulties resulting from occupation, then it is important to correct the factors which lead to the stiffening of the neck muscles and also to maintain the mobility of the neck joints and the elasticity of the muscles and ligaments. The following exercises should be done regularly:

(1) Drop the chin onto the chest and slowly stretch the head up and backward as far as possible. Repeat five times.
(2) Turn the head to the left, trying to get the chin as close to the shoulder as possible, and very slowly rotate to the right, looking over the right shoulder. Repeat five times.
(3) Without bending the head forward or backward, tip to the left side, trying to put your left ear on your left shoulder, and very slowly raise the head and tip to the right. Repeat five times.
(4) Drop the chin onto the chest and roll the head very slowly round in a clockwise direction, stretching the muscles as far as possible until you end up with your chin back onto your chest. Repeat in the reverse direction and then repeat this double movement five times.

These exercises are not physical jerks, so do them slowly, gently turning as far as is possible, and then try to force the movement just a fraction further. Repeat the exercises at least twice daily and also at any other odd times – when you are working, when you have been sitting in front of a computer, if you're stuck in a traffic jam. Just one or two of each movement will help to prevent the muscles of the neck and shoulders contracting and triggering off the symptoms of the stiff neck.

Tennis elbow

This is the most common condition caused by overuse of, and repetitive small traumas to, the elbow. It does in fact often occur in tennis players, but it may also be the result of any racket game and most other sporting activities that involve repetitive use of arm movements. It can also arise in people doing unaccustomed things, for instance painting and decorating; woodwork, especially prolonged use of a screwdriver; and I've even seen one patient who went on a brass-rubbing holiday and came back with tennis elbow. The pain is caused by inflammation of the tendons at the end of the large muscles which are attached to the outside bony surface of the elbow joint. This inflammation occurs as the result of overuse, unaccustomed movement or, frequently, poor techniques.

The immediate treatment should be rest and ice packs for the first 48 hours (the frozen pea treatment is ideal). Thereafter alternate hot and cold packs should be applied for ten minutes two or three times daily.

Osteopathic manipulation often provides the most successful form of treatment for this irritating condition. Rehabilitation and re-education are of great importance in overcoming the current injury and preventing repeated episodes. If the cause has been one specific racquet game, then close attention should be paid to the technique of playing and particularly the type of racquet used – weight, size, grip and materials used in construction. Increasing the size of the grip, reducing the weight and reducing the tension in the strings are all often helpful, as is a change to a fibreglass or composition racket which is able to absorb more impact through its frame and handle.

Improved muscle tone will protect the muscle joint from future injury and this can be achieved by a combination of isometric and normal exercises. Many enthusiastic games players would rather continue their game than give up because of tennis elbow. For these people the use of a properly designed, non-elastic elbow brace which is worn during playing and fits tightly around the muscles just below the elbow joint will provide considerable relief and will enable continued enjoyment of your game.

In practice I see many patients with tennis elbow and they often become quite depressed by this nagging and long-lasting condition. The normal orthodox treatment which usually ends in the use of steroid injections is not satisfactory and, in fact, repeated use of steroids can weaken the ligaments and make further, more serious injury highly likely.

Acupuncture is extremely effective in relieving the acute inflammation of the condition, and gentle massage using lavender oil will stimulate the circulation and encourage healing. It is always worth taking a short course of vitamin and mineral supplements, using those indicated in the treatment of arthritis.

Whiplash injury

This is an injury to the ligaments, muscles and vertebrae of the neck and is caused by a violent backward movement of the head. This type of injury is most frequently caused by rear impact car accidents. The violent forward thrust of the vehicle causes the head to be thrown backwards on the shoulders with great momentum. Normally the injured passenger has not had the time to prepare their muscles for the impact and consequently there is no restraint of movement. Muscle fibres and ligament insertions can be torn and damage to the bony structure of the spine can also occur. At the very worst this can result in severe injury to the spinal cord, possible fractures of the vertebrae, and even paralysis.

The fitting of head restraints to car seats minimises the risk of this type of injury, but only if they are properly adjusted. Head restraints should be in such a position that they make firm contact with the back of the head when the passenger or driver leans back in the seat. Unfortunately the common practice of using these restraints as neck rests and positioning them too low down in fact dramatically increases the risk of serious injury.

Ideally head restraints should be fitted to both front and rear seats wherever possible, and they must be easily and quickly adjustable, so that they can be arranged to suit the height of every individual driver or passenger. The point of contact between the head restraint and the head should be level with the ears and no lower.

Provided that there is no fracture of the vertebrae or serious involvement of the spinal nerve or roots, then manipulative treatment is the ideal form of therapy for these injuries. Gentle manipulations to correct small subluxations of the intervertebral joints are very effective. Mobilisation, massage and remedial exercises will do a great deal to restore normal movement as soon as possible and to alleviate sometimes longstanding pain which, untreated, may well become a chronic and disabling factor in the victim of a whiplash injury.

It is important to realise that the symptoms of a whiplash injury may not occur for some weeks or even months after the original accident. I recently saw a fit, healthy and athletic young man who started developing pains in his arms, hands and fingers some six months after being involved in a car accident. Although he suffered broken ribs and severe cuts and bruises in the accident, he did not feel any pain in his neck and this was not examined at the time of the injury. Anyone involved in a car accident with a sudden impact should see an osteopath as soon as possible after the accident in order to ensure that no damage has been done to the structures of the neck.

Respiratory problems

Asthma

Asthma is a condition which produces paroxysms of breathing difficulties together with wheezing. This is the result of the narrowing of the bronchi due to muscle spasms. This in turn increases the effort of breathing, making it very difficult for the sufferer to breathe out.

Asthma can start at any age but it is most common in small children or in middle age. Childhood asthma occurs in allergic individuals who produce antibodies to commonly encountered allergens. These stimulate the production of excessive quantities of histamine, which triggers the muscle spasm in the bronchi and is also responsible for the excessive production of mucus. It is the effort of pushing used air out of these constricted tubes, together with the added obstruction of mucus, that produces the characteristic wheezing sound of the asthmatic.

Asthma frequently goes hand-in-glove with eczema and hay fever and small children who develop the condition are likely to have had eczema as babies and to develop hay fever as they get older. There is very often a familial history of allergy.

Allergenic material is usually inhaled with the air and it is most commonly in the form of organic substances like pollen, particles from feathers or animal skins – especially dogs, cats and horses – or fungal spores. The faeces of the house dust mite contain one of the most powerful of all allergenic substances and this unavoidable little creature is present in all homes – even the cleanest. Asthmatic attacks may also be triggered off by foods and chemicals, the most likely being dairy products, eggs, wheat, yeasts and fish, together with many of the artificial food colourings, flavourings and preservatives. Of particular importance are the group of salicylates which are widely used in the food processing industry, especially for colouring foods aimed specifically at the child's mind.

Tobacco smoke, dust, cold air, exhaust fumes, chemical fumes, chest infections, sudden physical exertion, emotional stress, or even the effort of laughing can all trigger asthmatic attacks.

The successful treatment of asthma must be approached in a holistic way. Whilst there is no doubt that many of the modern broncho-dilator drugs dispensed in their convenient and effective

109

pressurised inhalers have done a great deal to ease the lot of the asthma sufferer, much more can be done by combining the best of complementary therapies with orthodox medicine. In this way it is often possible to avoid prolonged use of steroid medication since, although these drugs can be life-saving during an acute episode, their long-term use, if taken by mouth rather than inhaled, can cause extremely serious side effects. However, inhaled steroids are a vital part of treatment and are extremely safe.

The first step is to establish whether or not there are dietary causes of the illness and this can be done by following an exclusion diet (see Food allergies, page 269). Start by eliminating the most obvious substances previously listed.

In practical terms there are things which should be done to improve the environment in which the asthmatic lives. Bedrooms should not contain fabrics, carpets or rugs which can harbour the dust mite and other irritant particles. Floor coverings should be of lino or plastic tiles. Pillows, duvets and mattresses should be filled with synthetic materials, and the room should be vacuumed daily, including the mattress, and all surfaces where dust can collect should be wiped with a damp cloth before going to bed. The house dust mite thrives in warm damp conditions, so bedrooms should be kept cool and dry. Central heating which switches on in the early hours of the morning creates currents of air which waft the particles of allergenic material into the air which are then inhaled by the sufferer.

Asthmatic children should always be encouraged to take up some form of musical wind instrument and they should be encouraged to swim, as this is an excellent form of exercise for the development of the rib cage and all the secondary muscles of respiration.

There should be absolutely no smoking in the home of an asthmatic. Many asthmatic children feel deprived because they are not able to keep dogs, cats, rabbits, guinea pigs and other furry animals. This can be overcome by encouraging them to keep fish, lizards or snakes.

Most children do grow out of asthma but it is essential that every possible step should be taken to maintain their physical structure as normally as possible during the course of the illness. This will prevent the later development of physical changes like pigeon chest, spinal curvatures and reduced lung capacity.

Acupuncture treatment can be of great help in this condition and the acupuncturist will use the traditional meridian points to stimulate the flow of energy and help to relieve the bronchospasm.

Homoeopathy is particularly beneficial to the treatment of asthma but should not be undertaken on a self-help basis.

Osteopathic treatment offers considerable benefits. Manipulative treatment will help to improve the movements of the rib cage and consequently improve the volume of air which the sufferer can push in and out of his lungs. In addition, regular osteopathic treatment will help to prevent the postural abnormalities which so commonly develop in asthmatic children. Teaching the patient correct breathing exercises should also be part of the osteopathic treatment.

The overall naturopathic approach is to improve the nutrition of the patient, reducing the amount of dairy produce, increasing the amount of vegetables, fresh fruit and salads, and encouraging the consumption of fairly large quantities of fresh garlic (which can be taken as capsules).

Asthma is another of the conditions in which the ideal form of treatment is a combination of orthodox and complementary therapy. There are some practitioners, particularly homoeopaths, who would insist that patients stop all other medication before starting on homoeopathic treatment. This should never be done with asthmatics, particularly children. An acute asthmatic attack can be fatal and you should never change your own or your child's asthma medication without first consulting the doctor who is looking after you. In combination the different branches of medicine can work together and often produce dramatic results in the alleviation of this most distressing illness.

Bronchitis

In this condition the tiny airways of the lungs (the bronchi) become infected, usually following another infection such as a heavy cold or flu. This infection lowers the body's natural resistance and bacteria are able to multiply in the lungs, causing local irritation of the mucous membranes. These then produce more mucus which in turn becomes infected, producing a nasty cough, temperature, breathing difficulties, and thick greenish-yellow sputum.

Chronic bronchitis is the result of long-term irritation of the lungs, most commonly by cigarette smoke. Again the bronchi produce large quantities of mucus which does not become infected but forms an obstruction in the passages through which the air has to pass. Over a long period of time this loss of airway becomes more and more severe until in the end the patient will suffer chronic and permanent disablement. The only remedy is to remove the irritant substance, and patients who are not prepared to give up smoking and take better care of themselves by avoiding other irritants as far as possible have a gloomy outlook.

Regular inhalations with Climarome, and avoiding sudden changes of temperature, exhaust fumes, bonfires and going out in the fog, will all help. Above all, you must give up smoking and you must prohibit all smoking in your own home environment. Take as much care as possible not to catch a cold since this will inevitably lead to an infection of your already damaged lungs.

111

Homoeopathic treatment with aconite and pulsatilla is helpful, together with herbal treatment using a hot infusion of equal quantities of white horehound, hissop and amber flower. Three tablespoonfuls taken every two hours is recommended.

Excluding all dairy products from the diet will help to reduce the amount of mucus which your body produces, and regular osteopathic treatment to improve the mobility of the rib cage and the consequent efficiency of the whole breathing mechanism is extremely important.

A daily dose of 1 gm of vitamin C will increase your body's resistance to colds, especially during the winter.

One of the greater problems for the chronic bronchitic is that this disease is self-perpetuating. Because physical exertion is very difficult, the sufferer tends to become more and more sedentary, seldom venturing further than the garden gate, if that far. This lack of physical exertion promotes even less efficient breathing and allows the affected areas of lung tissue to grow. It is most important that the bronchitic keep as mobile as is humanly possible and he should be encouraged to take as much gentle exercise as possible. Repeated short walks, if the weather is suitable, or one or two minutes of regular exercise, even if done in your chair by the fire but repeated every hour, will help to stimulate lung function and circulation.

Catarrh

Catarrh is the excessive secretion of mucus from the membranes of the nose, throat, sinuses and from the upper part of the respiratory tract. Large amounts of mucus may be produced as a result of allergic reactions such as hay fever and perennial rhinitis, but it can also be produced following a simple cold. Repeated episodes can lead to chronic catarrh and the so-called 'post-nasal' drip which is responsible for irritating, persistent and recurrent bouts of coughing.

As a result of the excessive mucus blocking the sinuses, they may become infected, causing severe headaches and acute pain both above and below the eyes. Catarrh may also lead to ear problems, particularly in children when they are more liable to middle ear infections.

Many sufferers from this condition treat themselves with over-the-counter decongestants. The long-term use of these is not to be advised, since they can cause further irritation of the mucous membranes and lead to a rebound effect, hence aggravating the underlying condition.

Steroid nasal sprays may be prescribed for particularly severe inflammation of the membranes and these can be extremely effective. They are only recommended for short-term use since prolonged use of these substances can lead to thrush infections of the nose, throat and mouth.

It is most important to avoid inhaling irritant substances. Don't smoke, or spend much time in smoke-filled atmospheres. Avoid strong smells like paint, creosote, pungent air fresheners, and other toxic fumes. Follow the advice given under Asthma for keeping potential allergens out of your bedroom. If you do have thick catarrhal congestion, do not attempt to blow your nose too hard as this only forces the mucus down the Eustachian tube into the middle ear, and do blow one nostril at a time. It is a good idea to raise the head of your bed by about four inches (a brick under each castor at the head end of the bed is about the right height and the castor will fit neatly into the hollow of the brick). This encourages the mucus to drain better and prevents the post-nasal drip that causes chest infections. Regular inhalations with Climarome and a light application over the breastbone at bedtime will help to keep your passages clear.

Acupuncture is effective against catarrh since it is able to stimulate the flow of mucus and can also be used as a preventive measure. Massaging the acupressure points shown in the diagram below will also produce good results.

Osteopathic treatment to encourage drainage of the sinuses through massage and manipulation of the neck will promote

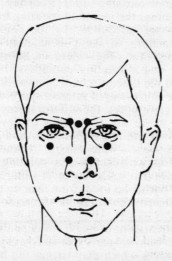

Acupressure points for the relief of catarrh. For
acupressure instructions, see caption on page 94

improvement and you should also take two Kwai garlic pills three times daily.

The homoeopathic remedy Nat. Mur. can also be used and a sensible wholefood diet excluding dairy products and eating small quantities of the starchy and sweet foods is extremely important.

An extremely effective treatment which I have used for well over twenty years is also worth trying. Using bottled beetroot juice available from most health food stores, you should mix one-third of beetroot juice with two-thirds of tepid water in a shallow dish. Put your nose in the mixture, close one nostril and sniff through the other so that the beetroot juice goes up your nose and into the back of your throat, then spit it out through your mouth. I know it sounds disgusting, but after the first sniff it's really quite easy. Repeat three times with each nostril and do it once a day or twice if your catarrh is extremely persistent. Beetroot juice is a mild astringent and will help to cleanse and wash out the nasal passages. Do remember not to use your best hanky for the next hour or two but stick to paper tissues as beetroot juice leaves permanent stains.

A daily dose of 500 mg of vitamin C and 40 mg of vitamin B6 should also be taken.

Hay fever

Everyone knows someone who suffers from hay fever – the running eyes, the blocked nose, the incessant sneezing from early spring to late summer. We are surrounded by the unfortunate sufferers. These allergic reactions to the pollens from flowering plants, grasses, trees and all the other allergenic substances make for a really distressing and disrupting condition. It so often affects children at around the time of school examinations and frequently interferes with the enjoyment of summer sports and pastimes.

To all intents and purposes, the sufferer seems to have a common cold. And whilst there are techniques of desensitisation which sometimes help, they are not without risk, and particularly where the sufferer is sensitive to a wide range of irritants the treatment is a long-drawn-out affair with usually disappointing results.

There is no doubt that some hay fever sufferers respond well to the elimination of particular foods from their diet. Commonly these may be dairy products, wheat, red meats and some of the artificial food additives.

The successful treatment of hay fever depends firstly on dietary change. It is worth following an exclusion diet by cutting out all the likely food substances which may trigger the hay fever and then adding them back one by one.

Acupuncture can be successfully used to reduce sensitivity to allergenic substances, but this is best done some weeks before the start of the particular patient's hay fever season.

Homoeopathic treatment with arsenicum album, euphrasia or allium oepa is recommended, together with large doses of vitamin C, up to 500 mg six hourly during acute episodes and long-term doses of vitamin B complex, 300 iu of vitamin E and 200 mg of bioflavonoids taken daily.

Keeping doors and windows tightly closed, avoiding going out when the pollen count is high, and the use of electrostatic air filters at home will all help. In addition, rinsing the eyes with distilled water and sniffing cold water through the nose will help to wash away irritant pollens and provide instant, if temporary, relief.

Sinusitis

Sinusitis is caused by inflammation of the mucous membranes that line the sinuses, which are the air spaces in the skull over and under the eyes. As with catarrh, sinusitis may be the result of an excessive production of mucus caused by irritation of the membranes, particularly as a result of allergy, or it can follow an infection such as flu or a heavy cold. Chronic sinusitis is usually caused by continuous irritation – by smoking, irritant fumes, hay fever, other allergies or food intolerance, especially to all dairy products. It can also be the result of polyps, small growths in the nasal passages.

Acute sinusitis can make you feel quite ill. High temperature, headaches, pain, loss of sense of smell and taste, and the discharge of thick foul-smelling yellow mucus from the nose and throat are all symptoms of this distressing complaint. Secondary infections are also common, especially of the chest and the middle ear, and this is particularly so in the case of small children. Nose drops, nasal sprays, decongestants and, especially in children, repeated doses of antibiotics, are the normal course of treatment. However, although these do help to relieve the symptoms, they do little about the underlying cause. Repeated courses of antibiotics are never a beneficial course of action. The long-term use of nasal sprays and inhalers may lead to damage of the delicate mucous membranes, causing a rebound sinusitis and aggravation of the original condition. In the absence of obvious allergy like hay fever, or asthma, one of the commonest factors causing this recurrent problem is an intolerance to milk and milk products. Many children respond well to the removal of all dairy products from their diet and this is particularly true for breast-fed babies whose mothers consumed large quantities of cow's milk. Reducing the mother's intake of cow's milk will reduce the incidence of catarrh and sinus problems in her baby.

Naturopathic treatment is extremely effective. A 48-hour fruit, vegetable and salad diet excluding all root vegetables, bananas, beans, and the removal of all dairy products, is the first step towards the resolution of sinusitis. Relief may also be obtained by mixing one eggcupful of beetroot juice (obtainable from your health food store) with two eggcupfuls of tepid water in a shallow dish. Put the nose in the mixture and, blocking one nostril, sniff up the other so that the liquid passes through the nose to the back of the throat and is then spat out. Three sniffs through each nostril, morning and evening, will provide relief for most sufferers.

As with so many respiratory problems, smoking is a key factor in this one. The effects of passive smoking, that is, the way inhaled smoke can infect non-smokers in the same environment, can be quite dramatic. Children brought up in a smoking home are twice as likely to suffer from ear, chest and sinus infections as children brought up in smoke-free homes.

Acupressure to the points shown in the diagram can produce considerable relief, and manipulative treatment to the neck and soft tissue massage to the neck and shoulder muscles, together with massage of the sinuses, encourages drainage.

Regular doses of Kwai garlic and 500 mg of vitamin C daily are nearly always helpful and the use of zinc tablets, particularly Zinc Cold, is a measure that I have found particularly helpful.

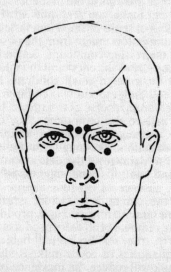

Acupressure points for the relief of sinusitis. For acupressure instructions, see caption on page 94

It is most important that you avoid flying if you have severe sinus problems or ear ache. Although aeroplane cabins are pressurised, they are not kept at the same pressure as ground level, consequently the difference in pressure can cause damage to the ear drum, especially in infected children.

Tonsilitis

This is an acute infection of the tonsils and is normally caused by streptococcus bacteria, although it may sometimes be caused by virus infections. Invading bacteria are trapped by the tonsils and killed, thus being prevented from reaching the lungs, but during this process the tonsils themselves may become inflamed, enlarged and infected, leading to a temperature, swollen glands, swollen adenoids, and the inevitable sore throat.

Tonsilitis is commonest in school children when they are first exposed to the myriad of bacterial and virus infections carried by other infants. It frequently leads to middle ear infections and when they are infected the tonsils become very enlarged and red, and may become covered in yellow spots.

Soft soothing foods such as ice cream, jelly, plenty of drinks and a warm environment are the basic needs of a child with tonsilitis, though if there is severe infection or middle ear complications, antibiotics are sometimes prescribed.

Happily, it is now less common to remove tonsils and adenoids as a routine procedure, but in children who do have recurrent episodes with severe infections, and especially when this affects their schooling, surgery may be indicated.

A cold compress round the neck, large quantities of diluted pineapple juice and extra vitamin C will help children to recover more quickly and in any case most children grow out of recurrent attacks by the age of 10 or 11.

During acute episodes gargling with an extract of red sage (half a teaspoon) to a cup of warm water several times daily will soothe the discomfort. Homoeopathic treatment with belladonna and a 24-hour fast on diluted pure fruit juices, vegetable juices and water, followed by 48 hours on fruit, salads and vegetables, will speed the recovery.

Problems of the heart, blood and circulatory systems

Anaemia

Anaemia is the name given to the illness in which the ability of the blood to carry oxygen to the cells of the body is reduced. Anaemia is caused either by bone marrow failing to produce enough red cells, the excessive destruction of red cells, or loss of blood, which can either be sudden, as in the form of injury or a haemorrhage, or it can be gradual through heavy menstruation, gum or bowel disease, or even piles.

The most common medical causes of anaemia are iron deficiency, vitamin B12 or folate deficiency (B12 deficiency causes pernicious anaemia), vitamin C deficiency or thyroxine deficiency.

The typical symptoms of anaemia are fatigue, lassitude, breathlessness, dizziness, headaches, insomnia, pallor (especially of the mucous membranes), palpitations, loss of appetite, and even pins and needles. In all forms of anaemia it is essential to establish the exact cause before commencing treatment, since there is no point in increasing the intake of iron if the patient is regularly losing blood, or if the body's own mechanism is destroying the blood cells. However, once a diagnosis is established, all forms of anaemia are best treated by improving the overall nutrition of the patient in addition to specific therapy indicated by the diagnosis. Pernicious anaemia is treated by injections of vitamin B12 as this has no effect on the condition when taken by mouth.

Careful attention to a good balanced diet should provide adequate iron and vitamins to ensure that anaemia does not develop, but there are periods when the body demands extra iron and folic acid, especially when children are growing, during pregnancy and in old age. At these times additional organic iron should be taken together with vitamin C in order to avoid possible problems.

Parsley, watercress, chickweed and dandelion leaves are rich in iron and should be included in your daily salad. Elderberries can be mixed with apples and blackberries since they are also rich in iron. Both comfrey leaves and stinging nettle leaves are rich sources and can be chopped and infused to make a tea. The general diet must contain ample quantities of iron-rich foods – liver, kidney, bread, wholegrain cereals, pulses, dried apricots, beef and molasses are good sources. All the leafy green vegetables, peanuts, almonds, tomatoes, yeast and vegetable extracts are rich in folic acid, whilst all animal proteins, especially offal, contain vitamin B12. But folic acid is easily lost in cooking and it is important to save your vegetable cooking water and add it to soups and gravies.

The absorption of iron is greatly helped by vitamin C, so always eat salads or citrus fruits when consuming iron-rich foods. It is also true that the body's ability to use iron is interfered with by caffeine, so avoid coffee, strong tea, chocolate and all the cola drinks.

Careless vegetarians, and particularly vegans, are at great risk of becoming deficient in vitamin B12, so it is very important for these people to take supplements; 25 mg of iron three times daily together with 2 mg of copper each day and 100 mg of vitamin C with each dose of iron will help to ensure that your body is absorbing as much as possible. A regular dose of 200 iu of vitamin E should also be added to any other medication.

Angina

This is the classical heart condition which results in pain in the chest and the left arm occurring during some form of physical exertion. The pain is caused by insufficient blood supply flowing to the muscles of the heart, which in turn is brought about by a narrowing or obstruction in the coronary artery.

The pain most commonly occurs across the front of the chest and behind the breastbone. Patients often describe the feeling of a large heavy weight pressing down on their chest. In many cases there is no sharp pain but feelings of discomfort often described as indigestion. These feelings can radiate into both arms, though more commonly it is the left arm which patients complain of, but it can also radiate upwards into the angle of the jaw, the side of the neck or into the shoulders. Symptoms are always precipitated by some physical exertion and this can be made worse immediately after eating or in extremely cold climates. A few moments' rest is usually enough to relieve the symptoms and the patient can carry on with his activities. But emotional stresses and conflicts are a frequent cause of acute attacks of angina and should be avoided.

In addition to the normal medication prescribed by the doctor, it is vital that the sufferers take regular gentle exercise and avoid emotional stresses. Overwork, overcommitment and a general lack of leisure are other important factors. It is also vital that angina sufferers should be encouraged to lead as normal a life as possible and should not allow themselves to be turned into invalids. With very few exceptions, most sufferers can continue in their normal occupations by making simple adaptations to their lifestyle.

In a small percentage of patients suffering from angina the condition is so severe as to prevent the patient from leading a normal life. In these cases surgical intervention may be necessary, and the most common procedure is that of a coronary artery bypass operation in which a piece of vein from the leg is used to divert blood around the obstruction in the coronary artery. A growing number of cardiologists are now in doubt as to the advisability of this procedure, since other less invasive and more holistic approaches to the disease are producing results which are as good as those from surgery.

Manipulative treatment to the area of the spine between the shoulder blades and to the joints and muscles of the rib cage can be of help in the treatment of angina. By improving the flexibility of the rib cage and the vertebral joints to which it attaches, it is possible to improve breathing and thereby increase the oxygenation of the blood.

Acupuncture is extremely useful in the treatment of angina and there are also good self-help points illustrated in the diagram (page 122). Herbal teas, especially chamomile and lime blossom, should be taken instead of tea and coffee, and homoeopathic treatment with cactus grandiflora or aconite can also be used.

It is very important for the patient to learn some form of relaxation therapy. Meditation, yoga and any one of the autogenic techniques for relaxation can all be tried.

Large doses of vitamin E are essential and should be taken regularly, starting at 800 iu per day, plus concentrated fish oils which will help the action of the vitamin E.

Angina is one of the commonest diseases of civilisation and is related to all the other heart and circulatory diseases. It is a preventable condition, but even if you have it, you can do much by altering your lifestyle to minimise the effects of angina and to reduce the possibilities of this illness totally disrupting the life of yourself and your family. (See Blood pressure, page 124 and Heart disease, page 126.)

Atherosclerosis

This is the name given to the disease in which atheroma, a cheese-like waxy substance, is deposited in the walls of the arteries. It occurs in all the large and medium arteries and particularly the coronary arteries supplying the heart muscle and the cerebral arteries supplying the brain. Over prolonged periods of time these fatty deposits block up the blood flow and, rather like putting your thumb over the end of a hosepipe, this causes the blood pressure to

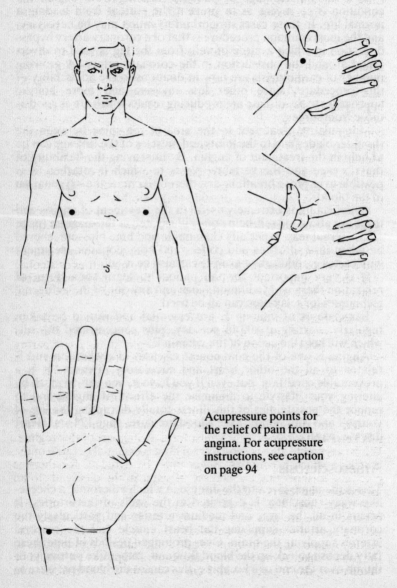

Acupressure points for
the relief of pain from
angina. For acupressure
instructions, see caption
on page 94

rise. It also increases the chances of clots forming in arteries. When the arteries affected are those that supply the arms and legs, they cause pain and swelling and, because the blood supply to the extremities is reduced, even minor accidents may lead to serious complications as the wounds will not heal and may even become gangrenous.

Twenty per cent of all deaths are caused by narrowing of the arteries which supply the heart. These deaths are needless since there is no doubt that atherosclerosis is yet another of the diseases of civilisation. Younger and younger members of our society are beginning to show signs of this illness. During the Vietnam war young American soldiers of only 18 years of age were found to have considerable deposits of fatty substances in the arteries supplying the heart. On a recent visit which I made to Harvard University Medical School, Professor Sacks told me that there was no doubt that the seeds of coronary artery disease are sown in childhood and some research workers even believe that it can begin during pregnancy as a result of the lifestyle of the mother.

This is undoubtedly a condition that can be avoided and one for which the only successful long-term treatment is modification of diet and lifestyle.

Smoking increases your chances of this disease by up to five times and cigarettes are the prime factor. Excessive quantities of alcohol raise the amount of fat circulating in the blood, and in susceptible individuals high intakes of animal fats, sugar and caffeine are all seriously linked with the disease.

A sedentary job and a lack of exercise combine together to increase your chances of atherosclerosis as well. At Harvard Professor Sacks has carried out large-scale studies comparing vegetarian and meat-eating populations. His conclusion is that a totally vegetarian diet results in much lower levels of blood fats than a meat-eating diet. I always recommend my patients with heart disease to switch to a vegetarian diet, and to reduce drastically their intake of dairy products, substituting vegetable oils, particularly linoleic and fish liver oils, especially those found in herring, mackerel and sardines. Fibre must form a vital part of this regime. Whilst vegetable fibre is good, cereal fibre is essential because of the mucilage which it contains. Sugar must be avoided, for there is evidence to show that an increase of sugar in the diet leads to an increase in the levels of cholesterol.

Women over the age of 35 who smoke and take the oral contraceptive are in a very precarious position. Their chances of getting heart disease are dramatically increased. In addition to the dietary factors, it is important to add some natural supplements to the food intake. A multivitamin and mineral supplement should be taken every day together with 1 gm of vitamin C, 200 iu of vitamin

E, 20 cc of linseed oil and 30 cc of lecithin. Ginger is effective in reducing the level of blood cholesterol and in preventing the formation of blood clots. Use it as a condiment and add it to all sorts of dishes, both sweet and savoury. Naturally, fried foods should be avoided. Garlic and oats also play a key role.

Relaxation exercises, biofeedback and autogenic training which teach patients how to cope better with stress; changes of work and domestic lifestyles to avoid unnecessary stresses, and a very sensible, very gradual and very gentle progression of aerobic exercises two or three times weekly: these will all improve the situation. The sensible management of this life-threatening disease is a rewarding experience, particularly for the patient. People are often able to recover their zest for living and, as long as they maintain careful control of their eating and living habits, they can look forward to a gradual return to normality.

Arteriosclerosis

This condition is one of the normal ageing processes which affects us all. The walls of the arteries become hard and rigid as a result of degenerative changes leading to deposits of calcium. It is frequently the result of high blood pressure and is often used incorrectly to describe atherosclerosis.

There is no specific treatment for this condition, although long-term therapy with high doses of vitamin E, 500 iu daily, may help to alleviate some of the symptoms. It is important for anybody with this condition to do everything possible to reduce the level of their blood pressure. See Blood pressure.

Blood pressure

The pressure of the blood in your circulatory system is a key measurement in knowing the state of health of your heart, veins and arteries. This pressure can vary enormously from moment to moment and day to day, depending upon what you are doing. In a normal healthy individual the pressure rises with physical exertion and falls at rest. One of the key measurements of fitness in athletes is the time which it takes for the pulse rate and the blood pressure to return to normal after severe exercise.

Serious problems can arise when your blood pressure becomes abnormally high or abnormally very low. One isolated abnormal reading is fairly meaningless but consistently abnormal readings are cause for concern.

High blood pressure (Hypertension)

A person is said to be suffering from high blood pressure when the measurements which are made exceed 149/90. The lower reading is in fact the more important, since this shows the minimum pressure of blood within the arteries. If this becomes consistently raised, the arterial walls become damaged and this can produce heart disease, angina and atherosclerosis. It is also possible for the small arteries in the brain to rupture under the strain of raised pressure, causing strokes.

High blood pressure can be caused by some diseases, particularly those of the kidney, the thyroid gland and gout, whilst obesity, oral contraceptives and a diet high in salt and saturated animal fats are often contributory factors. Smoking is the commonest single cause of high blood pressure.

In civilised Western society hypertension is the result of many different factors. Our diet, excessive alcohol, nicotine, stress, marriage difficulties, money worries and the strains of living in a competitive and frequently aggressive society, all play their part in the origins of this disease.

Complementary therapies, especially naturopathy, have been so successful in treating this problem that more and more of my colleagues in the orthodox medical profession are adopting techniques which we have used for the past half century.

A normal drug treatment for high blood pressure does nothing to remove the underlying causes of the disease, but merely uses drugs to control the problem. When blood pressure is exceptionally high these drugs are lifesavers, but the complementary use of drug therapy and naturopathy is a combination which reaps the highest rewards for the patient.

The first step is to make the necessary changes to lifestyle. You must learn some form of relaxation technique – biofeedback, autogenic training, yoga and meditation are all helpful. Reduce your intake of animal fats, alcohol and caffeine and especially nicotine. This is of the utmost importance. The ideal diet is that of a demi-veg – that is to say, cut out all meat and meat products but eat fish and modest amounts of poultry. Regular exercise which is aimed at increasing fitness is a major key to dealing with this problem on a permanent basis. Any form of regular aerobic exercise, brisk walking, swimming, cycling or any vigorous sport will increase the efficiency of the circulatory system. This enables the heart to pump a larger amount of blood with each beat. This training of the heart muscles produces rapid benefits. If you can reduce the heart rate by five beats per minute, you will cut down the number of beats your heart has to make each year by 2.5 million.

Osteopathic treatment can also be of considerable benefit. Improving the posture, improving breathing and teaching muscle relaxation techniques are all fundamental.

Herbal treatment with nettle tea, garlic and rutin and dandelion coffee to help increase the function of the kidneys should also be administered. Regular massage and the feelings of deep relaxation which this induces is also highly advisable.

Low blood pressure (hypotension)

There is a widespread myth that low blood pressure is a common and serious problem and that it causes all sorts of discomforting symptoms. Dizziness, fatigue, constant feelings of tiredness and general lack of energy and fitness are all attributed to this condition by patients who consult me in the belief that they suffer from low blood pressure. The fact of the matter is that low blood pressure hardly ever causes symptoms. Quite the reverse, in fact: it is a positive health advantage, since it relieves the heart of considerable strain and allows a far greater degree of reserve in the case of emergencies.

The one symptom that can be caused by this condition is that of postural hypotension. Rapid changes of position such as from sitting to standing, or lying to sitting, produce a sudden fall in blood pressure that lasts seconds. There is a temporary lack of blood to the brain cells and this can produce feelings of giddiness or faintness, but the blood pressure soon returns to normal and the symptoms are transient.

Occasionally drugs used for treatment of high blood pressure can reduce the level so much as to cause low blood pressure. This is easily remedied by reducing the amount of drugs taken.

The only time when low blood pressure is a serious problem is after an extreme and sudden loss of body fluids, during surgery, after severe injury which causes haemorrhage, or after prolonged bouts of vomiting. This sudden loss of fluid can cause shock, a drastic fall in blood pressure, and the risk of damage to the kidneys.

Low blood pressure can be treated with ginseng and a wineglass full of beetroot juice taken three times daily.

Heart disease

The commonest cause of premature death in the Western world is one form or another of heart disease. For the most part these early deaths are preventable and many of those that do occur are self-inflicted.

The whole question of heart disease and its relationship to cholesterol and high-fat diets has become a controversial subject. But, whilst it is certainly true that there are some people who naturally produce more cholesterol in their bodies than others, it is my strongly held belief that diet and heart disease are directly linked to one another. Angina, heart attack, coronary artery disease, diseases of the heart muscle, diseases of the heart valves – these are all more common in people who have higher levels of blood cholesterol than normal. Consistent high blood pressure, obesity, stress, smoking, alcohol and lack of exercise are common factors in people who suffer early heart attacks.

In spite of the controversy and all those who argue against the involvement of diet and lifestyle in this terrible disease, to ignore the following advice is foolhardy. Many experts believe that it is the key to a healthy heart and there is absolutely no argument at all over the fact that it is generally a healthier way to live in any case. So what have you got to lose? You don't have to become a health food freak or an exercise addict, you just have to use a little common sense.

You are what you eat, and so is your heart. Cut down drastically on the amount of animal fat you eat. Watch out for the hidden fats in meat pies, tinned meats, pâtés and sausages. Increase the amount of wholegrain cereals which you eat. Wholemeal pasta, oats, beans, lentils and other grains, wholemeal bread, brown rice – all these will increase your fibre intake which is beneficial and helps lower cholesterol levels. Eat more fish and poultry. Increase the amount of vegetables, salads and fresh fruits. Try to have one-third of your daily food raw. Cut down the amount of sugar you consume, not only the amount you add yourself, but that which is added to manufactured products. Learn to read the labels, because you'll find sugar hiding itself in the most unlikely places.

Cut down on alcohol – a little is beneficial, a lot is not. Cut down on your caffeine intake. Substitute decaffeinated tea or coffee or herbal teas for some of those middle of the day cups at home or in the office. Take up some form of regular sport or exercise. If you haven't done it for a long time don't rush straight out on to the squash court. This could trigger off the heart attack which we are desperately trying to avoid. One cardiologist friend of mine strongly suggests that nobody over 35 should play squash unless they are playing at least three times a week regularly. Walk more, buy a bicycle, have an active sex life – this certainly promotes a healthy heart in more ways than one.

Do ensure that there is a cut-off line between work and rest. You need time to relax and some form of meditation or yoga can be extremely valuable. Above all avoid overcommitment. Learn to say no and make sure that you plan your time sensibly. This will drastically reduce the amount of stress which you place on yourself. Try to have a massage once a week – even the cardiac departments in some NHS hospitals are using this treatment for their patients.

Above all, be sensible, because making such a supreme effort to stay healthy that your life becomes a drudge and a misery is counterproductive. The key to being healthy is being happy, so incorporate these tips with your normal everyday lifestyle. Don't let them become an obsession, but don't turn your back on them altogether, since that puts you on the path to sickness instead of health. If you haven't taken any form of exercise since you left school or, naturally, if you have suffered any form of heart disease, do check with your doctor before taking up any form of strenuous exercise.

Regular doses of vitamin E (400 iu), 500 mg of vitamin C and a regular dose of vitamin B complex is a good basic regime. You should also make sure that you have a regular intake of fish oil capsules or regularly eat mackerel, sardines or herrings – at least twice a week. Above all, add lots of garlic. Many people with heart disease are also subject to feelings of profound unhappiness. Money, work or marriage problems, dissatisfaction, and often deeply suppressed anger and frustration can all have adverse effects on the cardiovascular system and some form of counselling or psychotherapy is of great importance, not only in the prevention of heart disease in these people, but also in helping them to recognise the problems and avoid danger in the future. As with all forms of heart disease, osteopathic manipulation can be of immense benefit in conjunction with all the other therapies.

Piles (haemorrhoids)

These are small varicose veins which appear in the lower part of the bowel (internal piles) or around the wall of the anus (external piles). The most universal cause of piles is constipation, since in order to pass a hard stool considerable effort is required and this raises the abdominal pressure. The pressure stretches the small blood vessels and it is this which produces the piles. Apart from constipation the habitual use of laxatives, obesity, long periods of standing or sitting, pregnancy and frequent anal intercourse are all important contributory factors.

Piles are normally painful and can cause intense irritation. If constipation remains untreated, passing a hard stool scratches the thin skin of the bowels and causes bleeding. Untreated this can lead to the gradual development of anaemia.

The discomfort can vary in intensity from simply a mild irritant to the most severe and distressing problem. Local anaesthetic creams and, if necessary, injection or even surgical removal are all used in the treatment of piles.

Piles sufferers must pay careful attention to their own personal hygiene, washing the anus carefully after passing a stool and avoiding sitting for long periods on the toilet. The habit of disappearing to the lavatory with a newspaper and a packet of cigarettes for half an hour each morning is a sure sign that piles will follow.

Ice packs applied directly to the anus are the surest method of instant relief in the most acute stages of the complaint. Local applications of distilled witch-hazel can be used frequently throughout the day and especially after passing a stool. The homoeopathic remedies hamamelis and nux vomica should be taken. Twenty five mg daily of vitamin B6 and extra iron, folic acid and vitamin B12 (especially if there is continual bleeding) must be added to the daily regime.

Piles can be prevented, and even when you have them, taking the right measures will help in the treatment. You must not get constipated, and this can be prevented by eating more high-fibre foods such as wholemeal bread, cereals, pulses, fresh fruit and vegetables, dried fruit, and, most importantly, increasing your fluid intake. (You should aim at an average of 3 pints of fluid daily.) Eat plenty of fibre which is high in mucilage – linseed and porridge are good examples.

Contrast bathing with hot and cold water and more exercise will also help, not only with the circulation, but also with the problems of constipation.

During pregnancy the correct diet, the avoidance of constipation, taking care not to gain excessive weight and regular exercise are important measures to prevent the formation of piles.

Varicose veins

Due to an increase in pressure in the veins, they stretch and this causes them to become varicose. They can occur in various parts of the body, especially the rectum (see Piles), but most commonly are found in the legs. The calf muscles act as a pump when they contract and this helps to return the venous blood against the force of gravity to the heart. The blood is assisted along its way by a series of valves within the veins and when, for one reason or another, these valves stop working properly, blood can collect in the veins, stretching the walls and causing this condition.

Varicose veins may run in families due to an inherited fault in the valve system, but frequently are caused by periods of long standing or sitting, especially on hard-edged chairs, or by pregnancy, chronic constipation, lack of exercise and obesity, all of which can contribute to the formation of varicose veins.

Swollen ankles, pains in the feet, ankles and legs, and the distorted protruding veins are all signs of this condition. In the early stages a great deal can be done to reverse the situation – improving the diet to eliminate constipation and obesity, avoiding long periods of standing or sitting without movement, not crossing the legs when sitting, contrast bathing of the legs in hot and cold water, regular exercise, especially walking, and a daily dose of

200 iu of vitamin E will all reverse the trend towards varicosity.

In the most severe cases varicose eczema may develop on the legs and this can result in varicose ulcers, which are extremely difficult to treat and can take a long time to heal. The use of honey as a treatment for varicose ulcers can produce excellent results. Apply on a gauze strip and keep in place with a bandage.

Herbal treatment with tincture of calendula rubbed over the veins three times daily and rutivite tablets together with homoeopathic arnica and pulsatilla form part of the treatment. Gentle massage rubbing upwards towards the heart, using fifteen drops of rosemary oil in three tablespoons of almond oil and a daily dose of 1000 mg of bioflavonoids with vitamin C and 10 mg of lecithin have all been found effective.

The treatment which I have used for many years with great success is as follows. Obtain two large plastic buckets from your garden centre. Also purchase a large bag of pea shingle from your local builder's merchant. Place about 4 inches of pea shingle in the bottom of one bucket. Fill this bucket with hot water, fill the other bucket with cold water and add to the hot water two teaspoons of Kneipp rosemary oil. Stand in the hot water, walking around and stomping your feet up and down on the shingle for one minute. Then transfer your feet to the cold water for fifteen seconds, then return to the hot water. Repeat this procedure for ten minutes twice daily, always finishing with the cold water and following with a good brisk friction rub with a coarse towel.

There is considerable evidence to show that varicose veins are yet another of the diseases of Western civilisation. Dr Denis Birkett, the world authority on bowel disease, has suggested that this condition is a direct sequel to a lack of fibre in our modern diet and the resulting constipation.

Skin problems

Skin (oily, spotty, open pores, etc.)

The outer layer of skin, or epidermis, serves as a protective barrier to guard more delicate tissues from injury. This hard outer layer is waterproof and is in a constant state of replacement by new cells growing from the bottom layer of the epidermis. The skin is constantly shedding the dead scales of the surface and new replacement cells move up from the growing layer to the outside in approximately three weeks. The deeper layer or dermis contains sebaceous glands which continuously secrete sebum, an oily substance which coats the skin, both protecting it and serving as a defence against bacteria. People's skin varies in the amount of sebum which it produces and it is this that decides whether you have dry skin, normal skin or oily skin. At around the time of puberty both boys and girls are producing more male hormones – androgens – and these stimulate the glands to produce more sebum.

Skin is richly supplied with sensory nerve endings which relay all the sensations of touch and feel to the brain. Pleasure, pain, itching, touching, heat or cold are all transmitted through the skin sensors. As well as being a huge area of sexual excitation due to the heightened stimulus of stroking and touching and the specific sensitivity of the erogenous zones, skin appearance is also an important sexual factor.

Many people, especially adolescents, who have skin problems, particularly eczema, psoriasis and acne, can tend to shy away from any overt sexual contact for fear of embarrassment. These feelings of shame or even guilt can also affect the work situation, especially if the job involves dealing with the public.

A range of differing problems can affect skin at different ages.

In babies and infants nappy rash may appear. This is caused by the skin bacteria reacting with urine to produce ammonia. This is very irritating and can form painful sores on the visible areas of the skin. Washing to remove all the bacteria is essential at every change of nappy. Some babies develop seborrhoeac eczema of infancy which can also affect the creases of the body which are not covered by the nappy area. It appears around the neck and under the arms and is often present with cradle cap. This condition is not true eczema and usually disappears completely. In the meantime, avoid all soaps and detergents and use only emulsifying ointments or aqueous cream for cleaning the baby. The old-fashioned remedy of zinc and castor oil cream is most effective and with care and scrupulous attention to the hygiene of the baby you can avoid the common occurrence of thrush which infects the rash.

Infantile eczema may also develop. (See Eczema, page 140 and Skin allergies, page 135.)

Every adolescent's nightmare is the spectre of acne. But it does affect almost every teenager during puberty because of the increased production of the male hormone androgen. (See Acne, page 134.)

In adult life a common problem that particularly affects women is that of stretch marks. These occur when there is any dramatic increase in body weight, stretching the skin and causing tiny cracks in the supportive structure. During pregnancy excessive weight gain should be avoided in any case for general health reasons, but also in order to prevent the residual stretch marks which will be left behind. This is particularly important for slim women as they have less skin to stretch to begin with, and any sudden rise in weight is likely to leave them with far worse stretch marks than those who are heavier to start with.

Vitamin E creams may help to minimise the effect, but nothing will remove the underlying damage to the skin structure. During pregnancy the extra hormones produced may improve acne and psoriasis, but eczema tends to get worse. The tiny blood vessels in the skin swell and can produce red marks and swelling of the hands and feet. The hormones may also stimulate the production of melanin in the skin, causing changes to pigmentation. Brown patches may become apparent on the face, but they will disappear much more quickly if exposure to sunshine is avoided.

Exposure to irritant chemicals both at home and at work can cause dermatitis. (See Dermatitis, page 139.) Protect hands from strong disinfectants, detergents and all washing powders, especially biological washing powders.

With age all layers of the skin become thinner. Elasticity may be lost and wrinkles become more prominent. Excessive exposure of the skin to sunlight and weather makes this ageing of the skin more noticeable on the face and neck. Due to the decline in hormone production with age, less sebum is produced by the sebaceous glands and the skin becomes much drier. Avoiding soaps and detergents can help.

Effects of sunlight

Too much exposure to sun without doubt hastens the ageing

processes of the skin and encourages the earlier formation of wrinkles. There is also a very definite link between sunshine and skin cancer. People who spend their lives working in the open air in hot sunny climates have a much higher incidence of skin cancer in old age, whilst those, especially blue eyed and fair skinned people, who spend most of their lives indoors at a desk and then spend three weeks of the year toasting themselves like chickens on a barbecue on a Mediterranean beach are much more likely to develop malignant melanoma in early adult life. How the sun affects your skin depends very much on your skin type (as distinct from the sun protection factor of the cream). The ability of your skin to become tanned depends on its classification:

Type 1 – never tans, always burns – red hair, Celtic
Type 2 – always burns, sometimes tans
Type 3 – sometimes burns, always tans
Type 4 – never burns, always tans
Type 5 – pigmented skin

Those who have type 1 skin must always use high factor protective creams or lotions as they are at risk of serious damage. Gradual exposure to sunlight in small, but increasing doses when you go on your holiday is the only way to avoid the severe discomfort of sunburn which can, at its worst, cause dehydration, sunstroke and serious illness, and at best peel off your skin, removing what little tan you have acquired so that you have to start all over again.

There are some people who have an allergic reaction to ultraviolet rays, in fact it can affect as much as 10 per cent of the population, women rather more than men. A rash of red spots normally appears during the evening after one or two hours of sunbathing or walking around in the sun. The rash can last up to ten days, but repeated exposure to sunlight reduces the reaction and, as the summer wears on, the rash will gradually disappear. In some cases only intense sunbathing will produce the rash, but that is enough to spoil your holiday. Some drugs and the effects of perfumes on the skin can increase the chances of allergy to sunlight.

There is no evidence to support the theory that taking vitamin tablets will either protect you from sunburn or promote tanning. Some of the suntan lotions contain extract of bergamot and, whilst these do increase the tanning effect of sunlight, they certainly increase the rate of skin ageing and may increase the risk of skin cancer.

The best method of preventing the occurrence of spots, pimples, boils and other infective skin blemishes is cleanliness. Skin may be cleaned with detergents, scrubs, lotions, gels, creams and soaps, all of which will remove the surface grease, dead cells and dirt. For most skins mild soap and water followed by thorough rinsing is sufficient, but for people whose skins are dry to start with, the soap may remove what little grease there is. In this situation a cleansing lotion or cold cream is a suitable alternative. Liquid soaps especially, since most of them contain detergents, are very drying to the skin. For this reason many bath products are not ideal ways of looking after your skin, particularly bath salts and bubble baths. Taking a shower instead of a bath and using natural bath oils will help to minimise the drying effect on the skin.

In principle, expensive does not necessarily mean better when considering cosmetics, skin lotions and cleansers. The basic ingredients are much the same for all products, and it is only that more expensive perfumes and 'nourishing' or 'regenerating' ingredients of dubious value have been added. Even many of the hypoallergenic creams contain lanolin, preservatives and colourings which may cause allergic reactions. Remember that the surface layer of the skin comprises dead cells and no amount of expensive potions will bring them back to life. The apparent benefits of these products arise from moisture being absorbed through the outside layer of the skin and swelling the tissues underneath, hence ironing out wrinkles and other blemishes. When this moisture is absorbed or lost through evaporation, the skin returns to its previous shape and texture.

Above all, you are what you eat and a poor diet will be reflected in a poor skin.

Acne

Eighty per cent of young people between the ages of 12 and 24 are likely to suffer from this unpleasant condition to a greater or lesser extent. During adolescence an increased production of the sex hormone androgen causes the sebaceous glands in the skin to produce larger quantities of sebum. The sebum makes the skin more oily and the sebaceous glands become blocked up, causing blackheads or whiteheads. These can then become infected, creating swollen, red and painful pustules. The infection is often spread by scratching the spots with dirty fingers. Acne usually occurs on the face, neck, back and shoulders and is often aggravated by emotional distress, anxiety and poor diet.

The first step in treatment is to improve the diet. Cut out fried foods, fatty foods, excessive amounts of sweets and chocolates, and reduce the amount of dairy products. Increase the amount of vegetables, salads and fresh fruit. Secondly, it is essential to keep the skin impeccably clean. Washing regularly with 'Simple Soap' and scrubbing the skin with fine oatmeal will keep it clear of infecting bacteria. Use natural yoghurt as a face-mask in the evenings and apply for at least 15 minutes. Be very careful with oily aftershave, colognes and cosmetics. Many young girls are tempted to cover their spots with makeup, which serves to increase the number of pores which get blocked and aggravates the condition.

A facial sauna which allows you to steam the skin is extremely helpful, and adding elder or marigold flowers to the water will increase the effectiveness. Distilled witch-hazel is an excellent astringent and skin cleanser. The homoeopathic remedies of heparsulphuris and silica will help to minimise the formation of pus and the development of scars.

Periodic cleansing diets for three days each month will also help. These should consist exclusively of salads, lightly cooked vegetables and raw fruit for two days, introducing grains and pulses on the third day. Hot and cold water alternately applied to the affected areas and followed by a brisk friction rub with a rough towel will stimulate the circulation and help the healing process.

Exposure to sunlight is always beneficial, but before using artificial sunbeds consult your practitioner for detailed advice.

Vitamin therapy is extremely useful. I recommend 2500 iu of vitamin A three times daily, 5 mg of zinc gluconate three times daily and, where the acne is worse around the time of menstruation, 50 mg of vitamin B6 daily for the week preceding the onset of the period and the few days during it.

Skin allergies

In addition to causing asthma, hay fever and a host of other allergic problems, the body's abnormal response to allergenic substances also frequently involves the skin. (See also Eczema, page 140 and Nettle rash, page 146.)

These allergic reactions involve the body's own immune system, which is the defence mechanism through which we fight infection. The body is able to identify foreign substances and instruct large volumes of white cells to collect at the sign of invasion and do battle. Sometimes this system goes haywire and the white cells overreact, causing more problems than the original invading organism or substance. In this situation the body's response produces allergic illnesses, and whilst in my practice I have come across some truly outlandish cases of allergy, there are groups of substances which are most commonly the cause of problems. Dust, pollens, metals (particularly nickel), cosmetics, lanolin, animal hairs, stings, bites and some drugs – especially penicillin and aspirin – are all frequently the cause of allergic reactions. Strawberries, shellfish and eggs, together with many of the food additives, especially tartrazine, sulphur dioxide and benzoic acid, can cause problems, as can the chemicals used in washing powders and soaps.

Cow's milk is probably the most widespread cause of allergic reactions throughout the world. Most of the populations of Asia and India are unable to digest cow's milk satisfactorily and this problem also frequently occurs in Europeans. Most widely affected are babies, and it has even been shown that breast-feeding mothers who consume large quantities of cow's milk can have an adverse effect on their babies. A common allergy which cow's milk produces in babies is infantile eczema.

Allergic reactions can sometimes be devastating in their effect, particularly those to insect stings and fish, with patients rapidly developing severe symptoms, particularly breathing difficulties which can prove fatal. Although it is possible to treat allergies with desensitising injections, this is a long, complex and unpleasant procedure, particularly if the patient is suffering from multiple allergies. Furthermore, it is not without hazard and it has been known for the treatment to produce severe shock in some patients. The sensible approach is to identify the allergen wherever possible and try to avoid it within the pattern of your normal lifestyle. This is easily done with some substances but much more difficult when one is dealing with pollens, fungus spores and dust.

Over the years I have become more and more convinced that there are three factors involved in these types of reactions. Firstly the allergy response itself. Secondly the question of intolerance, particularly of foods. This can produce symptoms similar to those of allergy but the response is not a true allergic reaction. Finally, mental and emotional stresses. There is no doubt that these play an important role, particularly in the allergic responses which result in skin problems. One only has to see how frequently these problems improve often dramatically during holidays, when exams are all finished, or on retirement. It is important to look into the psychological background of people suffering with these problems since some form of psychotherapy, hypnosis or relaxation therapy can often be a useful extra dimension to other forms of treatment.

Boils, carbuncles and styes

When bacterial infection attacks hair follicles or sweat glands the result is usually a boil, which will normally come to a head within a few days and burst, releasing the bacteria and white cells in the form of pus. The application of hot poultices speeds up the process but you should never squeeze a boil or try to lance it with an unsterile needle. In most cases boils do not need more treatment than simple hygiene, but very large painful boils in sensitive areas of the body like the face, buttocks or thighs may need to be treated with antibiotics, or even be lanced under sterile conditions.

136

A boil that develops in the follicle of an eyelash is known as a stye, and a collection of boils developing in adjacent hair follicles becomes a carbuncle.

Many people have bacteria on the skin which cause no problems. However, if you become run down, or a patch of skin suffers constant friction, or you scratch a pimple with dirty hands and fingernails, or even when the skin is already broken because of dermatitis, scratches or other abrasions, boils may develop more easily.

People with diabetes are much more likely to suffer from boils since the level of sugar in their blood can become raised to abnormally high levels.

Some boils are much more painful than others, particularly those in the nose or ears, and boils on the face, especially in the area between the nose and the eyes, need special treatment, since it is possible for the infected pus to travel inwards and cause serious infections. Simple boils, whilst a nuisance, are no cause for concern, but frequently recurring boils, carbuncles, boils associated with high temperatures or occurring in the very young or very old need specialist attention and should not be interfered with without advice.

A hot kaolin poultice will help to bring the boil to a head more quickly, or a poultice made with powdered slippery elm mixed with boiling water into a thick paste can also be used. Once the boil has burst, use the slippery elm as a cold poultice until healing is well under way. Homoeopathic treatment with belladonna or silica will also be an advantage and a daily intake of 50 mg of zinc until the boil has healed is recommended.

Stimulating the skin with alternate hot and cold friction rubs and attention to a well-balanced diet rich in vegetables, salads and fruits and low in high-sugar and high-fat foods is essential to prevent recurrent attacks of boils.

Calluses

These are thickened hard layers of skin which may develop on the palms of the hands, folds of the feet, heels or sometimes on the elbows and always result from repeated friction due to occupation or ill-fitting shoes. Severe callusing of the skin on the heel can sometimes lead to deep cracks and fissures which are extremely painful and may easily become infected. They should be treated by soaking the feet in warm water with a few drops of olive oil, followed by gentle rubbing with a smooth pumice stone and the liberal use of pure lanolin (some people are allergic to lanolin and a small test patch should be done first to see if there is any adverse reaction). Initially the lanolin should be put on in thick layers,

137

covered with a pair of old socks just prior to bed. Do this three times a week. As the calluses recede you can use smaller quantities rubbed well into the skin every night and use a thick application once weekly until the calluses are completely gone.

While the skin is cracked and open it is important not to go barefoot and to pay careful attention to regular washing and drying of the feet and frequent changes of socks.

Corns

Keratin is a form of protein which increases the strength of the protective covering of the skin. A corn is a skin lesion caused by pressure on the skin's surface stimulating the production of excessive keratin. Badly fitting shoes bought for fashion rather than comfort are the commonest cause of corns. They can occur on the upper surface of the toes, on the outer edges of the feet or, if you have hammer toes, they will appear on the tips of the toes since with this problem your body weight is not distributed through the pads of the toes, but directly below the end of the nail.

If you have corns, take them to a chiropodist. Trying to get rid of them on the cheap by using proprietary plasters, paints or patent corn cutters usually results in the top surface being removed and this is not sufficient. Furthermore, your chiropodist will be able to advise you as to the cause of your corns and suggest preventive measures.

Treating corns without changing the type and fit of your shoes is a total waste of time.

Corns can become a serious problem for the elderly. Keeping active is vital if they are to keep their heart, lungs and circulation functioning efficiently. Painful feet prevent them from going out and walking and should be attended to without delay.

Corns can give you back ache. Yes, it's true. Not so long ago I saw a patient who had been having treatment for a bad back for well over twelve months. Doctors, physiotherapists, orthopaedic surgeons, acupuncturists and even an osteopath had failed to give her more than temporary relief. We soon discovered why. She had a large corn on the outside edge of her right foot. This was so painful that she walked with a pronounced limp. The limp upset the natural weight distribution throughout her spine. This distorted her posture, which in turn placed severe stresses on the ligaments on the opposite side of her back.

No amount of treatment would have helped this lady, but sending her to a chiropodist cured the corn and the back problem in one fell swoop.

Taking care of your feet, removing areas of hard skin with a smooth pumice stone after soaking in hot water, applying regular quantities of lanolin rubbed well into the skin of the feet, keeping the toe-nails properly cut, and, above all, wearing good shoes and good socks – avoid those made from synthetic materials as far as possible – all these measures will help to ensure you don't suffer from corns. If you are unfortunate enough to have one, applying a dressing of crushed garlic over the corn does help to relieve the pain, and the garlic oils soften the skin.

Dermatitis

Contact dermatitis is the commonest form of skin allergy. It usually arises in the most sensitive areas of skin – the backs of the hands, the eyelids, the inside of the wrists, the nape of the neck and at the hairline are all regular sites for this distressing condition. The skin itches and then reddens. It frequently becomes scaly and dry. Finally, blisters can form which break and weep. The skin can become very puffy and swollen, and although this type of dermatitis can appear after one exposure to an allergenic substance, it is usually the result of months or even years of continual irritation by the suspect substance.

Hair dyes, perming lotions, a multitude of chemicals, rubber, antibiotics, perfumes, preservatives and, most frequently, nickel, are the commonest causes. Costume jewellery, which is frequently made from rolled gold over nickel-containing alloys, can trigger dermatitis on the fingers, earlobes, neck and wrists. The patch around the belly button is usually caused by the metal studs on jeans, whilst patches between shoulder blades come from the hooks and eyes on bras and on the inside of the wrists from the metal buckles on watch straps. I have often noticed patches of dermatitis on women's thighs and these correspond exactly to the fastenings on suspenders. These are normally rubber-covered nickel. Do look for plastic zips, press studs, hooks and eyes and other fastenings if you have sensitive skin.

Perfumes are a great hazard. Nearly all toiletries and cosmetics are perfumed. Deodorants, talcum powders, shampoos, hair creams, shaving creams, cosmetics and nail varnish can all be villains in this detective story. The allergic effect of the substances in perfumes is considerably increased on exposure to sunlight. It is essential that you do not use any form of perfume or per-fumed cosmetics when sunbathing or when using sunbeds. In fact, before doing either, a bath or shower is an extremely good idea.

Patients with dermatitis on the hands are frequently advised to avoid contact with detergents, washing up liquids and other chemicals and to do this they should wear rubber gloves. Unfortunately this is a real catch 22 situation, since these people will almost certainly be just as sensitive to the rubber.

Even natural products are not totally innocent in this area. Contact with poison ivy, primroses or chrysanthemums and even touching fish, eggs or almonds, and especially coming into contact with animal skin and fur, can all produce an allergic reaction leading to dermatitis.

Unfortunately the skin reaction is not confined always to the area which has been touched. After repeated irritations the dermatitis can spread to areas of the skin far removed from those in contact with the aggravating substance.

The only certain cure for this condition is prevention. You must identify the substances which aggravate your skin and avoid them. Not so long ago I saw a child who had an extremely sensitive skin, but her problem had been well under control for some time. Her mother was meticulously careful to avoid all the known allergens. One morning she woke up with her back and chest covered in a bright red dermatitis. It looked exactly as if she was wearing a red vest and I asked her mother if she had changed her washing powder, since we had gone to great lengths to find one that did not aggravate the child's skin. It transpired that the manufacturers had changed the washing powder, and after I mentioned this particular story on my Body Talk radio programme, more than two thousand letters arrived within a week from people suffering the same problems. The manufacturers of the washing powder denied absolutely that the changes they had made could have had any effect on the skin. In fact they even produced an eminent dermatologist who appeared on the radio show. In spite of denying any responsibility, within a few weeks the old original formula was back on the market side by side with the new one, which was biological.

To relieve extreme itching, a cream or gel of aloe vera together with the homoeopathic remedy graphites or Rhus. Tox. will be found helpful. Occasionally, food allergies can be responsible for aggravating dermatitis and it is worth eliminating cow's milk and its related products from the diet or even trying an exclusion diet for a few weeks.

Five hundred mg of oil of evening primrose, 2500 iu of vitamin A, and a good vitamin B complex taken daily will help to strengthen and protect the skin.

Eczema (See also Dermatitis)

Those unlucky people who suffer from asthma, hay fever and eczema are described as being atopic. These unfortunates may suffer from more than one of the problems and they may also have to endure urticaria (nettle rash). This last can be the result of food or drug reactions, or contact with plants such as chrysanthemums or primroses. Atopic eczema is nearly always a familial complaint and although different generations may suffer different symptoms, a history of atopic illness usually spreads throughout the family tree.

Eczema may frequently be triggered by stress, but the major cause inevitably is allergy. This allergy, particularly in babies and small children, is less likely to be a contact problem and much more likely to be a reaction to foods, medicines or inhaled substances. For this reason the normal patch tests for allergies are little more than useless in determining the allergic factors at the root of infantile eczema. More recent tests, using applied kinesiology, electrical testing or ACR (auricular cardiac reflex), are a much more promising method of investigating food allergies. Though these techniques are derived from modern methods of acupuncture and manipulative therapy, there is a growing number of doctors specialising in ecological medicine using these methods. Sadly, the mainstream of orthodox medical opinion shows little interest in techniques which involve concepts based on the complementary medicine theories. Beware the extravagant claims of some allergy clinics.

Infantile eczema can appear between the ages of 3 months and 12 months and can then persist well into the late teens. The skin is dry, the patches of eczema are also dry, red, itchy, sometimes even weepy. In severe cases the skin splits and bleeds. The frenetic scratching often leads to scarring and continual rubbing of the itchy patches causes a thickening and ridged appearance to the skin. The areas most commonly affected are the folds behind the joints of the knees and elbows, and the face, particularly around the eyes and mouth. In black and Asian children with eczema the skin may look raised and pebbly. Other factors which can also affect eczema are very cold windy weather, emotional stress, or contact with some synthetic fibres, wool or nylon. The hot dry air produced by central heating or the cold dry air produced by air conditioning can make eczema far more uncomfortable.

There is a growing body of evidence to show that food allergies are frequently an aggravating cause in a large percentage of atopic children with infantile eczema.

A food exclusion diet is the first step. The commonest implicated products are eggs, cow's milk and many of the artificial colourings, flavourings and preservatives. While there seems to be a lower occurrence of infantile eczema in breast-fed babies, breast-feeding mothers who themselves consume large quantities of cow's milk are more like!y to have babies with eczema.

Baths should never be taken too hot. Keep them cool with non-detergent essential oils or emulsifying creams for cleaning the skin. These also help to reduce irritation. Most bath salts, bubble baths and other bath additives contain chemicals which dry out the skin and can be very irritating. Swimming in the sea frequently improves eczema, particularly in conjunction with sunshine. Chlorinated swimming pools can be very irritant and children must shower immediately they come out of the water.

The normal medical treatment with steroid ointments can provide temporary relief, but long-term use can cause damage to the skin and if these creams are used together with dressings which cover the ointment this can encourage the absorption of the steroids into the bloodstream, which can have serious general side effects. Coal-tar ointments and antihistamines are frequently prescribed to reduce the itching and help encourage sleep, but sadly many of the medicines prescribed for children contain the very colourings and flavourings which may aggravate their condition.

With small babies you must keep fingernails very short to minimise the damage done by scratching. It's useful to keep thin cotton gloves on the baby's hands at night. You can prevent babies and smaller children removing these by taping round the wrist of the glove with sellotape. This must not come into contact with skin but should be stuck to the sleeve of the pyjamas. Do not ever use elastic bands to keep them on, as they can interfere with the circulation.

A diet which excludes the obvious possible allergens and is high in green leafy vegetables, root vegetables and fruit, provided it is not citrus fruit or acidic berries, will help. For the adult, avoiding excessive quantities of alcohol and caffeine can be beneficial. Some people with eczema respond well to a diet which excludes red meats, though this is not true for all sufferers.

Vitamin and mineral therapy is the same as that for dermatitis.

Disorders of the hair and scalp

Hair and scalp disorders crop up with monotonous regularity on the phone-in programme and in the correspondence which I get. People worry desperately about their hair and go to the most amazing lengths, to say nothing of expense, to try to prevent baldness, to restore hair growth, or to change their hair from straight to curly, or curly to straight. The majority of things which people do to their hair are at best useless and at worst damaging. Hair loss in young men can be a traumatic experience, in young women devastating. One young black patient of mine recently committed suicide. A tragic loss of a bright young girl. Why? Because in an effort to straighten her curly hair she damaged it so severely that it fell out, and she was unable to cope with the trauma of this awful experience.

There are all sorts of reasons for losing hair and for its varying condition. There are things you can do to improve the health of your hair, and these are on the whole simple, inexpensive and safe.

Baldness in men is a strong genetic characteristic. If your father or your mother's father went bald early, the chances are that you will go bald early. Male baldness is the result of hormone changes and none of the proprietary highly expensive preparations that are available on the market will prevent the genetic inevitability from occurring. In fact, many of these substances cause irritation to the scalp and can even result in dermatitis. One of the drugs used in the treatment of high blood pressure has been shown to stimulate hair growth, though only in very special situations. The application of this drug is very limited.

Women do lose hair as they get older and it may become very fine and thin, but they lose much less hair than men in their younger years. Most women suffer quite considerable hair loss within about three months of having a baby. Again this is the result of hormone changes, but the hair soon grows back again.

Radiotherapy, chemotherapy, serious illnesses and sometimes surgery can result in temporary hair loss and both men and women can suffer from alopecia. This is a condition in which small round circles of the scalp, or in men the beard, lose all their hair. Sometimes these small areas then join together, but this condition is best left well alone, since in time the hair will grow back.

If you suffer from severe dandruff, dermatitis of the scalp, or ongoing hair problems, it may be worth consulting a trichologist for advice and treatment for your particular condition. But the underlying message is that if you take care of your hair and take care of your health, you should avoid many of the problems that are so common today.

Choose your shampoo carefully. Do not use products which contain strong detergents. Wash your hair frequently. Try to avoid harsh bleaches and dyes. Don't perm your hair too often. Rosemary or nettle shampoos are excellent tonics for the hair, and rubbing some almond oil into the scalp before shampooing does prevent the scalp from drying out.

The homoeopathic remedy sepia is useful for hair loss and bryonia will help with greasy hair and kalicarbonicum for dry hair.

A really good massage to the scalp will stimulate the blood supply and improve the nutrition of the hair follicles. Once a fortnight carry out the following procedure. Wash the hair with your normal mild shampoo. Warm a little olive oil. (Do not put it in a pàn on the gas stove but place a bowl containing the oil into a larger dish of hot water until the oil is warm.) After rinsing the hair, massage the warm olive oil into the scalp; using the tips of the fingers and applying firm pressure, massage for at least five or six minutes. Wrap a towel around the head and leave the oil on the scalp for at least half an hour. Wash again, using the minimum amount of shampoo, and rinse thoroughly.

If you suffer from dandruff you can use natural yoghurt as a conditioner. Wash the hair, rinse, apply the yoghurt and rub it well in, leaving on for at least fifteen minutes. Rinse out and wash the hair again with as little shampoo as possible.

It is important to realise that hair and scalp problems may be a sign of some other underlying illness. This is particularly true of nutritional deficiencies and modern methods of hair analysis are extremely useful in determining the levels of minerals, trace elements and toxic elements in your body's system. If you have an ongoing hair or scalp problem, do seek professional advice from a naturopath. In any case, a good balanced healthy diet is the first step towards healthy hair.

Vitamin E, manganese, zinc, copper and iron are all important for the health of your hair. In addition, some extra vitamin A and wheatgerm oil will also be of benefit.

Don't forget that ringworm, a fungus infection, can cause small patches of baldness and this is common in children. Ringworm must be treated with fungicides. The head louse is also a frequent cause of hair and scalp problems. Look out for these in children. Head lice are increasingly common and are no respecters of cleanliness. In fact the head louse probably prefers short clean hair to long, lank, dirty hair.

Using medicated shampoos is not sufficient to eliminate the head louse. A fine comb is the louse's worst enemy. Since the louse tries to grip on to the hair, the comb pulls its legs off and thus kills the louse. Contrary to popular belief, you cannot get lice from other people's hats, combs, hairbrushes, towels, mats in gymnasiums, swimming pools, or the back of the bus seat. The only way you can catch lice is by head to head contact. So be alert for the louse; it affects small boys and girls equally, although as the children get older it seems to prefer the female heads as the hair is denser and easier for it to get a grip on. If you suspect your child has lice, do get proper advice so that the problem can be totally eradicated, as it is a very distressing thing for the children and can eventually make them quite unwell.

A final word for women. Anaemia is a problem which can cause hair loss. This is particularly true in women who have heavy periods and who may be deficient in iron. So if you have heavy periods, or if you start losing some hair, do get professional advice and in the meantime take extra iron and vitamin C.

Herpes (cold sores, genital herpes and shingles)

Cold sores
Caused by the virus herpes simplex, cold sores are highly infectious.

By the age of five most children have picked up this virus from an already infected person. The virus remains dormant in nervous tissue until it is stimulated by some other illness – colds, sore throats, high temperatures, and particularly unaccustomed exposure to sunlight. Skiing or seaside holidays are a frequent cause of the eruption of cold sores.

An uncomfortable irritation starts in the skin around the lips. This is followed by the eruption of tiny blisters which gradually become covered with a crust. After about 10 days the crust dries and the sore usually heals. But as long as the affected area remains moist, the sores are highly infectious.

Genital herpes

This is also caused by the virus herpes simplex, although a different strain. The first attack of genital herpes is nearly always the most uncomfortable. It is commonest in young people and appears as small painful blisters in the genital region, buttocks and thighs. Genital herpes is also highly infectious and is easily spread during intercourse. Often the initial infection arises after oral sex with a partner who has cold sores.

If a pregnant woman suffers an attack of genital herpes this can have serious repercussions for the baby, particularly if the attack is very near to the time of delivery. Some authorities consider that this is sufficient cause to justify delivery by caesarian section in order to prevent the baby becoming infected with the herpes virus during its passage through the birth canal.

There is a definite link between genital herpes and cancer of the cervix, and any woman who has suffered from this problem should have a cervical smear test yearly.

Shingles

This is caused by the virus herpes zoster, the same virus that causes chicken pox. And like the cold sore virus, it remains dormant in nervous tissue. Most commonly shingles affects the nerves running between the ribs, commonly on one side, although it can appear on both sides together.

Shingles is probably the most painful form of herpes. The pain can begin up to four days before the appearance of any visible signs and then tiny incredibly painful blisters appear all at once. They finally dry up after about fourteen days. Occasionally shingles can affect the trigeminal nerve on the side of the face, which can lead to infection of the eye.

One of the worst problems with shingles is that the acute pain can persist for weeks, months and sometimes years after all visible signs of the rash have gone. Shingles is usually seen in older people and is not very common under the age of 40.

145

Herpes infections are highly contagious. If you have cold sores do not kiss other people, especially babies and young children. Do not indulge in oral sex. If you have genital herpes, avoid any form of sexual relations, hetero- or homosexual, until at least ten days after all the sores have dried up and the scabs have gone. The use of a contraceptive sheath can afford protection to both partners against recurrent reinfections. (This is also true of other sexually transmitted diseases.)

If you suffer from cold sores you must always use a high factor sunscreen when on holiday. This is particularly true if you are skiing, mountain climbing or boating.

The residual pain of shingles is not only excruciating but can be highly depressing. This pain is resistant to even the most powerful of analgesics, but I have found over the years that the use of acupuncture as an analgesic can be extremely effective as a safe palliative measure.

Distilled witch-hazel will help to dry up cold sores more quickly and the homoeopathic remedies of Nat. Mur. and Rhus.Tox. will help.

At the first sensations of skin irritation, rub the lips with a slice of lemon or dab with lemon juice.

Daily doses of l-lysene at 1 gm per day, together with a high potency vitamin B complex, can be useful in the treatment of all types of herpes and the residual pain of shingles.

There are some new anti-viral drugs now available. It is not thought to be sensible to use these powerful drugs in the treatment of minor herpes infections, but they can be extremely valuable in the treatment of more serious problems.

Nettle rash (hives or urticaria)

This is an acute allergic skin reaction which produces burning and irritating pale coloured weals which look just like those caused by stinging nettles. Nettle rash can come up on the skin where it has been in contact with an allergenic substance or all over the body if it is the result of food allergies. Apart from the obvious stinging nettle, other plants can cause similar problems, particularly poison ivy, chrysanthemums and primroses. Shellfish, ordinary fish, milk, nuts, wheat, strawberries, eggs and even chocolates are amongst the more usual foods that produce nettle rash, although individuals may have quite idiosyncratic allergies.

In some susceptible individuals stress can play a major part in triggering attacks of nettle rash, but the permanent solution lies in avoiding substances which are known to be the triggers.

If you suffer from nettle rash, make sure that you do not wear synthetic materials next to your skin. Cool baths and liberal

146

applications of calamine lotion will relieve the acute irritation. An infusion of marigold flowers (calendula) and taking echinasia tablets will also help, and large doses of vitamin C, up to 1000 mg daily, are a good idea.

Psoriasis

Psoriasis is a very common illness, estimated to affect approximately two million people in England. It is caused by skin which grows too rapidly in some places and forms thick inflamed red patches covered by a silvery scale. Psoriasis can develop on damaged areas such as elbows and knees and can also appear on the site of other injuries. The body can be affected anywhere and there are some patients who are covered in red scaling skin. If the scalp is badly affected the scaling can produce hard lumps and flaky dandruff. Occasionally psoriasis may be associated with a form of arthritis, especially on the toe and finger joints. When the condition becomes severe it can be disfiguring and cause considerable emotional stress to the patients who suffer anguishes of embarrassment. Not unnaturally they are wary of going swimming or sunbathing and this can become a very real emotional problem, particularly for young women.

When the skin becomes very thickened, inflamed fissures can develop which are painful and sometimes begin to bleed.

The normal age of onset of this condition is between fifteen and twenty-five, but it can come at any age from earliest childhood to old age. It is not infectious and you can't give it to anybody else. We don't know exactly why patches of psoriasis start, but it can appear after some illnesses, particularly severe sore throats, after surgery, after taking some prescribed drugs, and often after acute sunburn. There do seem to be family connections in this problem and most patients will have at least one close relative who also suffers with psoriasis. Generally speaking, most sufferers improve during the summer months and get worse again during the winter.

Unfortunately there is no magic answer to this condition. There are treatments which alleviate the symptoms and these work by slowing down the growth rate of the skin and clearing up individual patches. Some of the medicated ointments do help, but they smell awful and are very messy to use. Steroids are sometimes prescribed but should be used with great care, because long-term use can damage the skin still further.

Never allow yourself to become sunburned as this will make your psoriasis worse. Even so, gradual and careful exposure to sunlight can be very beneficial and I am never surprised when my patients come back from a summer holiday with their skin looking marvellous. Ultraviolet lamps do help but must be used with great caution. Excessive exposure to ultra-violet light can increase the chances of developing skin cancer in later life.

It is always worth making dietary changes for the treatment of this condition. They may help and they can't possibly hurt, since all the dietary changes recommended are those compatible with sound nutrition. (See Allergies, page 269.) As with so many skin conditions, stress can be an important factor in psoriasis. Psychotherapy, relaxation techniques, biofeedback and autogenic training can all help to improve the body's eliminative functions, whilst acupuncture and hypnosis help to control the dreadful itching which this condition causes.

Two tablespoonfuls of almond oil containing one drop of lavender oil and two drops of calendula oil, thoroughly mixed together, should be massaged into the affected areas every evening. Regular treatment with vitamin A supplements is an essential part of treatment. Do not exceed the recommended doses as too much vitamin A can cause other problems.

Athlete's foot and ringworm (tinea)

Both these conditions are caused by a fungus infection which invades the skin. Ringworm – it gets its name from the round raised patches which look just like a worm – is found in the groin, beard and scalp, whilst athlete's foot appears between the toes. Ringworm can cause hair to fall out, leaving small round bald patches both in the beard and on the scalp. Tinea, to give it its Latin name, is highly contagious and spreads by physical contact. For this reason it is common in young men engaged in contact sports such as rugby, judo or wrestling. It also occurs on horses and cattle and is a frequent hazard for people who have close contact with these animals.

Local applications of antifungal medications usually work, but persistent ringworm may need oral treatment.

As with any fungus infection, personal hygiene is vital. Bed-linen, towels and flannels should be washed separately in normal temperature washing powders. Low temperature washes will not be sufficient. If you have athlete's foot, make sure that you only wear cotton socks and wherever possible avoid wearing tights or stockings. Avoid wearing shoes made of synthetic materials as these encourage sweating and produce conditions in which the fungus can thrive. Change your socks at least twice a day, washing the feet at the same time. Dry between the toes very carefully, but avoid excessive rubbing as this will damage already sensitive skin. Local treatment with calendula ointment is soothing and a very light dusting with arrowroot powder will help to avoid excessive moisture.

Cataracts and drugs

New evidence shows that many drugs increase the sensitivity of the skin and eyes to ultraviolet radiation. Professor Donald Pitts, of the University of Houston, specialises in visual science. He told me that young people are getting cataracts, and of course the amount of skin cancer has grown dramatically in recent years. It is not just sunlight, but all the ultraviolet from computer screens and fluorescent lights that is worrying.

On his list of dangerous drugs:

- **Oral contraceptives.**
- **Tetracyclines** – antibiotics often used for acute chronic bronchitis.
- **Griseofulvin** – prescribed for fungal infections of skin and nails.
- **Chlorathiozides** – diuretics (water pills), long-term use is common.
- **Benzodiazepines** – minor tranquillisers (like Valium and Librium).
- **Sulphonamides** – often prescribed for urinary infections.
- **Psoralens** – used to treat psoriasis; often present in suntan lotions and Earl Grey tea.
- **Phenothiazines** – major tranquillisers (like Largactil).
- **Sulphonylurea** – oral diabetic drugs.

If you are taking any of these drugs, extra care regarding ultraviolet light is vital.

Glasses and contact lens manufacturers Cooper Vision produce a unique material, called Permaflex, which protects the eyes in a way ordinary sunglasses can't. But you can only get these glasses and lenses with a prescription in Britain.

A good start might be for manufacturers to supply a pair of protective goggles with every VDU.

New research indicates that eating foods rich in vitamin C and beta-carotene reduces the risk of cataracts in later life.

Problems involving the urinary and reproductive systems

Frigidity and impotence

These two problems affecting women and men respectively seem to be a growing concern. I see more patients with these problems, and receive more letters from the public about them, than ever before. Apart from the various factors described below, there is no doubt in my mind that a gradual decline in the quality of nutrition and the ever increasing stresses with which people live in our modern society are at the root of many of these psychosexual problems. Concern about the dramatic increase in sexually transmitted diseases, especially AIDS and herpes, role reversal in male/female relationships and worries about the overexpectation that surrounds so much of the sexual information appearing in the media today, all contribute to people's insecurities. These problems are by no means related only to the older section of our community and young people in the prime of life are afflicted with both impotence and frigidity.

Most sexual problems arise between couples, and when dealing with both frigidity and impotence, the problems cannot be dealt with in isolation. The couple should consult a therapist together to achieve optimum results.

Frigidity

This lack of sexual enjoyment and stimulation is sometimes the result of long-standing illness. It can be caused by irritation, discomfort or dryness of the vagina, which occurs quite commonly after the menopause.

A lack of sexual desire is frequently the result of tiredness, having small children, or even the direct result of careless stitching of the perineum following an episiotomy during childbirth. In this situation the vaginal opening is sometimes made too small, causing great discomfort to the woman.

Depression, anorexia, previously traumatic sexual experiences, recurrent cystitis or thrush may all also be factors to consider.

Whole books have been written about the psychological factors in these types of sexual disorders and the same is true of impotence. Once the possibility of specific physical causes has been ruled out, counselling or sex therapy is the treatment of choice.

Using a simple lubricant like KY jelly is an obvious but usually overlooked solution to any discomfort caused by dryness of the vagina.

Contrast bathing with hot and cold water can help to stimulate the circulation to the whole of the genital area and, naturally, a sound nutritional intake is important to maintain the integrity of all the mucous membranes.

Vitamin E taken at the dose of 200 iu daily and an overall naturopathic approach to the total health of the patient are also important.

Impotence

When a man is unable to ejaculate or maintain or even get an erection, he is described as being impotent. There are physical causes of this problem, for which there are now good treatments, but, in the majority of cases, it is psychological.

Impotence can be caused by some drugs, especially tranquillisers and those used to treat high blood pressure, excessive quantities of alcohol, or changes in the hormone balance. The mechanism which maintains the erection is dependent on an adequate flow of blood into the penis. Consequently, anything which interferes with the circulation can adversely affect the man's ability to have an adequate erection. Smoking is a prime example, since nicotine constricts the tiny blood vessels at the end of the circulatory system and men who smoke will have smaller erections than they would if they gave up. Enlargement or disease of the prostate gland can also cause impotence.

As with frigidity, stress, tension, anxiety and overexpectation can all be factors in this condition. A vicious circle ensues in which the stress causes impotence, which causes more anxiety, which causes more stress, and eventually chronic depression.

Psychotherapy is usually the treatment of choice for this problem, provided organic causes have been eliminated. Sex therapy with your partner, and under the guidance of a skilled practitioner, can produce dramatic benefits, but it does require time and patience.

5000 iu of vitamin A and 200 iu of vitamin E taken daily, with some additional zinc, will help and it is worth trying a short course of ginseng or guarana.

There are no magic aphrodisiacs, but looking after your diet, making time to enjoy your partner, and the use of relaxation techniques to help deal with your stress problems, should all provide beneficial results – but do not be impatient.

Kidney stones

Stones in the kidney can cause what is probably the most excruciating of all pain. Stones may be composed of uric acid, but more commonly they are either calcium oxalate or calcium phosphate. Repeated urinary infections, especially cystitis, can lead to infection of the kidney and make the formation of stones more likely. Since women are more prone to cystitis, they are more likely to contract this form of stone.

Most people do not drink sufficient fluid, and this leads to the urine becoming more concentrated. If this situation is aggravated by the overuse of saunas, or by occupations which involve considerable sweating such as bakery, glassmaking, steelworking or working in extremely hot climates, then the likelihood of stones is increased even more. Kidney stones can vary from tiny gravel-like grains to large 'stag horn' stones which can become lodged in the kidney.

Stones can cause damage to the structure of the kidney or the associated structures or in extreme situations can cause complete obstruction. If there is any sign of blood in the urine, or difficulty in passing water, you should consult your doctor immediately.

Kidney stones may have to be removed surgically, although new techniques using beams of sound waves which disintegrate the stone and allow the small particles to be passed avoid the necessity of major surgery and allow the patient to return home within a matter of days.

Complementary therapies can be used to treat kidney stones, but of course they are more effective in preventing a recurrence of stones in people susceptible to forming them.

Tea made from the herb parsley piert, commonly known as parsley breakstone, is an age-old remedy for this problem. Extract of dandelion is an effective diuretic, helping the body to eliminate urine. If you are prone to stones you must keep your fluid intake to a minimum level of 3 pints of liquid daily. A homoeopathic remedy, berberis, will help to relieve kidney pain and a large mixed salad should be eaten every day containing dandelion leaves, parsley and raw chopped leek.

Fifty mg of vitamin B6 and 300 mg of magnesium should be taken each day. You should avoid an excessive intake of high calcium foods, especially dairy products and foods containing oxalic acid, like spinach, beetroot, rhubarb and chocolate. Start each morning with a glass of warm water containing a teaspoonful of honey and a dessertspoonful of apple cider vinegar.

If you are on holiday in the sun or working in extremely hot conditions, you need to increase your fluid intake even more than the 3 pints recommended per day.

Menopause

The menopause is not an illness. It is a normal function of the human body and is the time when women stop menstruating. The age at which it occurs varies considerably, but as a rough guide it usually happens between 45 and 55.

Many women seem to be hardly aware of going through this menopause, but some suffer badly. Hot flushes, night sweats and a drying up of the mucous membranes in the vagina are common. A serious and often untreated side effect of the menopause is the gradual loss of calcium from the bones. This can lead to osteoporosis or brittle bones in later life and is preventable by taking the proper steps. There are drastic changes in the hormones produced by the body at this time and this is responsible for many of the symptoms, but psychological difficulties also occur which may be the cause of lack of sleep, depression, bad temper, repeated headaches and a general malaise. These problems also need to be dealt with and taking up yoga, learning relaxation therapy, or even some form of group therapy or counselling can be a great aid.

Hormone replacement therapy (HRT) can be the most successful way of dealing with severe problems with the menopause. It certainly reduces calcium loss and the modern techniques of using very low dose hormone pills are considered safe, but women receiving this treatment should have constant supervision and monitoring by their doctor.

To help with the stresses and tensions, make a mixture of equal quantities of pulsatilla, lime blossom and raspberry leaves. Add one teaspoon of this to a cup of boiling water. Stand for five minutes, strain, add honey and drink. Don't neglect your diet during the menopause. Ensuring a well-balanced food intake will improve your overall level of health and vitality. You should also supplement your diet with 100 iu vitamin E three times daily, and 50 mg B6, 200 mg of calcium, 100 mg magnesium and 10 mg zinc each day.

Premenstrual syndrome (PMS)

The premenstrual syndrome is a distressing collection of symptoms which produces physical, emotional and behavioural changes in millions of women during the few days just before the onset of their period. These changes affect all areas of women's lives and can be the cause of dramatic upheavals: failed relationships, broken marriages, distraught children, lost jobs, accidents and even criminal activity.

Estimates of the number of women affected vary between 40 and

70 per cent – and those who suffer are often condemned to spend a quarter of their lives in the most abject misery. Even women who have comparatively mild symptoms are likely to be 25 per cent less efficient in everything they do, at home or at work, for at least one week a month.

In spite of the size of this appalling problem, I have been horrified by the number of desperate women asking for my help as an alternative practitioner in overcoming the very real difficulties caused by PMS. Their stories were almost universally the same: repeated visits to doctors who seemed to care little and know even less, the inevitable prescriptions for tranquillisers, anti-depressants and sleeping pills, and the feeling that they were always treated as yet another neurotic female destined to limp through life supported by the crutch of behaviour-modifying drugs.

Alternative practitioners have long believed that there is a nutritional factor involved. Dietary improvements and supplements of vitamin B6 and zinc had produced good results in many patients. Yet there was not much scientific evidence to prove that some of the alternative ideas had any value. A few specialised doctors had done some experiments with their patients, but their good results do not seem to have found their way into widespread use by GPs. In spite of all the indications of things that might help, no serious, large-scale studies have been done.

Together with LBC and a women's magazine, I decided to try to find some vital answers, with the help of my listeners and readers. In response to an article in the magazine, nearly 2000 wrote in asking to join our special study, which was designed to look at the effects of simple changes in diet, together with a vitamin and mineral pill.

It is clear that a poor diet leads to lower levels of some of the essential nutrients, which in turn causes some of the worst symptoms. Sugar cravings, headaches and tiredness; poor excretion of sodium which is the cause of fluid retention and consequent bloating; over-indulgence of animal fats and dairy products, raising the level of calcium in the body, which adversely affects the magnesium balance and so the body's hormones; drinking too much tea and coffee, both of which interfere with its uptake of iron and zinc, and cause overstimulation of the brain and nervous system.

As you can see, much can be done to help the situation by improving the diet. However, there are occasions when a vitamin and mineral supplement, taken regularly, may be more useful. When the symptoms are severe, most women find it hard to make any extra efforts to take better care of themselves. Swallowing a pill is simple, and requires no additional shopping, preparing or cooking.

There are lots of pills on the market claiming to be 'the answer' for PMS. They range from the very cheap – not likely to be much help, as the quantities of vitamins and minerals are too low – to the very expensive, which contain a host of exotic ingredients with little relevance to the problem.

The ideal product seemed to be 'Magnesium-OK', which contains suitable amounts of the key substances: magnesium, zinc, selenium and vitamins B, C, D and E. At a dose of one pill a day it was simple and it's inexpensive. The manufacturers, Wassen International, agreed to supply the tablets and to fund the cost of the trial.

The experiment was designed and carried out with the help of a major university, and has been the first 'double blind crossover' study of this scale. The participants were screened to ensure that those included were as typical as possible of the population as a whole.

Of the 2000 women who filled in an initial registration form, some were excluded at this stage for reasons of age, other health problems, or because they were receiving other medical treatment. A second and detailed questionnaire was sent to the remainder. This gave us information about their general health, lifestyle, diet, smoking, alcohol consumption, exercise, menstrual cycle, age, height, weight and number of children.

This left 670 women to take part in our study. Each was asked to fill in a chart, recording the severity of their symptoms, weight and the day on which their period started. This was done every day for four months, during which time they were divided up into four groups.

Group A were given Magnesium-OK.

Group B were given a 'fake' pill that looked just like the real one – a placebo.

Group C got the real pill and a simple list of dietary changes.

Group D had the placebo and were asked to make the same changes to their eating habits as Group C.

The dietary changes we recommended are not hard to follow, and if you suffer from PMS you *should* give them a try:

(1) Cut down on your tea and coffee consumption. Try not to drink more than *two* or *three* cups altogether each day. Instead you should use herb teas, unsweetened fruit juices, or savoury drinks like Marmite or Vecon. Avoid cola drinks as they contain caffeine.
(2) Increase your consumption of wholegrain products – wholemeal bread, wholemeal pasta and brown rice. Use oats, barley, nuts, seeds, lentils and beans.
(3) Eat more fish (especially sardines, mackerel, tuna and salmon); more poultry and less red meat.

(4) Eat a salad each day, and plenty of green and root vegetables.
(5) Use *less* salt. Don't sprinkle it over your food, and put as little as possible in cooking. Avoid salty foods – crisps, salted nuts, bacon, kippers and the like.
(6) Cut down on sugar, especially the 'hidden' sugar in cakes, biscuits, sweets, chocolates and fizzy drinks.
(7) Keep alcohol consumption to a minimum.
(8) Watch out for the 'hidden' fats in meat products, and cut down a bit on all dairy products.

You may have cravings for all the wrong things just before your period. Try to resist, you may feel better if you can.
We looked at the ten most common symptoms of PMS:

(1) Feeling swollen and bloated.
(2) Loss of efficiency.
(3) Irritability.
(4) Weight gain.
(5) Difficulty in concentrating.
(6) Tiredness.
(7) Mood swings.
(8) Tension.
(9) Restlessness.
(10) Depression.

The first thing we found was a direct link between some of the symptoms, which seemed to occur in groups:

Numbers 3, 9, 7, 8 and 10
Numbers 2, 5 and 6
Numbers 1 and 4

In each group there was one symptom which was most significantly improved by the treatment: numbers 1 and 6 by the pill alone, number 8 by the pill and the improved diet. Bloatedness, tiredness and tension are the most easily identified in their groups, and so probably those in which changes were most obvious.

For all ten symptoms, the best improvements in four cases were produced by the pill, in four by the pill and the diet, and in two by the diet alone. There was not one symptom for which the placebo proved to be better than the other treatments. One fascinating fact to emerge was that those women whose diets were the worst to start with showed the smallest level of improvement. This is almost certainly because their bodies were less efficient at using the vitamins and minerals in the pill.

By the end of our study, those who had been taking the pill and following the dietary improvements, including those with bad eating habits, were showing signs of catching up.

In the case of the four symptoms where the diet and pill together proved most successful – weight gain, mood swings, tension and restlessness – the diet would have improved the overall vitamin levels and encouraged better digestion and absorption of the pill's contents. Improved eating habits could be related to all the changes for the better, and we know from the questionnaires that the women who took part in the trial had a higher than average awareness of healthier eating.

Over the course of this experiment the percentage improvement for all ten symptoms were:

The pill	56–78%
The pill + diet	47–94%
The diet	59–86%

Bearing in mind that a good, well-balanced diet is a more natural source of nutrients, one would expect it to be at least as good as the pill, if not more so. In reality, it seems that a good compromise is to make as much improvement in eating patterns as you can, and to supplement this with a suitable vitamin and mineral pill.

I certainly believe this to be the case, particularly for those of you whose diet is really poor to start with. In the long term, there are a host of other vital reasons for better eating. Living on a junk food diet and popping vitamin pills is not any kind of solution.

But, as our survey has shown, adding a simple, natural remedy to an improved diet, can help to overcome the misery of PMS. The long-term treatment is in your own hands. Eat well – feel better.

Prostate problems

The prostate gland is a part of the male reproductive system and its size and the secretions it produces are controlled by male hormones. The prostate can become infected, causing an unpleasant condition known as prostatitis. This is normally an infection which causes general malaise, some frequency of urination, and some discomfort on the passing of urine. It may also cause severe back pain. It is normally difficult to isolate a specific kind of bacteria but the prostate, although not enlarged, becomes extremely tender.

In older men, this gland can enlarge, when it causes pressure on the urethra (the tube connecting the bladder to the penis), which makes it necessary for the patient to pass urine very frequently. As the gland gets larger it can interrupt the flow of urine and this can make both starting the flow and indeed stopping it rather difficult. After stomach and lung cancer, cancer of the prostate is the third commonest affecting men. It is rare under 60, but when it does occur it can be the secondary deposits, particularly in the base of the spine, which produce the first symptoms, namely severe back pain. The enlarged prostate can be treated by surgery. This sometimes led to impotence after the operation, but new techniques avoid this problem.

Coffee, tea and alcohol will certainly aggravate an already enlarged or inflamed prostate gland. They should be avoided and the fluid intake increased. Contrast bathing of the whole pelvic and genital area with alternate hot and cold water night and morning will help to stimulate the circulation in the area and eating one ounce of pumpkin seeds daily helps to reduce the size of the prostate because of their high zinc content.

Two teaspoons of sunflower oil and 50 mg of zinc should be taken daily if you have prostate problems. I recommend my older male patients to take a preventive dose of 10 mg of zinc and two capsules of sunflower oil every day.

Thrush and cystitis

These are common conditions, causing untold misery and discomfort to millions of people, mostly women.

Thrush

This is an infection caused by the yeast candida albicans. Candida is normally found living quite happily with other bacteria and yeasts in our mouths, bowels, skin and other mucous membranes. When the natural balance of these organisms is disturbed, the number of candida cells multiplies dramatically, producing an attack of thrush. This frequently happens in the mouth, throat, around the anus (especially in babies), in the vagina, the urinary tract and on the head of the penis.

The contraceptive pill, antibiotics (especially when used over a long time), pregnancy, cystitis, chronic diseases, and general exhaustion or excessive stress leading to a lowered natural state of resistance, can all precipitate an attack of thrush.

In the mouth it shows as small white patches on the lips, gums, tongue and inside of the cheeks, which can be very uncomfortable. In the vagina, thrush produces intense irritation and quantities of unpleasant smelling white or yellow discharge. Where the penis is infected, the tip becomes inflamed, red and sore and there may be some discharge. Hands and feet are not exempt. The nails can be deformed and cuticles become damaged and painful. It is now recognised that thrush can sometimes cause a general and debilitating condition which produces symptoms of malaise, fatigue, depression, irritability, and flu-like aches and pains, which are often associated with food intolerances and caused by the candida organism affecting the whole body. The normal treatment using fungicides rarely succeeds in the long term, but alternative therapy can be of great help, together with things that you can do for yourself.

Thrush is highly contagious and easily spread by sexual intercourse. If you or your partner have this condition, both of you must be treated and you must abstain from sex until all the symptoms have gone. Stop taking the contraceptive pill. Wear only cotton underpants. Try to wear stockings, not tights. Don't use medicated soaps, disinfectants or bubble bath in your bath-water. Avoid very hot baths and excessive washing of the genital region. Once daily with warm water and 'Simple Soap' is enough. You must eat a carton of natural yoghurt each day and you should apply some natural yoghurt to the vagina morning and evening (using a tampon inserter makes this quite simple). Don't overexercise, because hot and sweaty bodies are ideal breeding grounds for the candida organism. For one month eliminate sugar, bread, mushrooms, tea, coffee, chocolate and alcohol from your diet. But eat as much as you like of fresh fruit, salads, vegetables, wholegrain cereals and garlic (if you're worried about the smell you can take Kwai garlic). You should take a yeast-free megavitamin B complex tablet every day and these are obtainable in all good health food stores.

Cystitis

This common bladder infection also causes great discomfort. Again it is seldom possible to identify a specific kind of bacteria causing it, but cystitis frequently occurs in conjunction with thrush and is more common in women than in men. Women often get this condition as a result of sexual activity (honeymoon cystitis), but it can also be a form of allergy. When it does occur in men it is normally the result of an inflammation of the prostate gland (See Prostate problems, page 158).

The classic symptoms of urinary frequency, scalding pain when passing urine and pain just above the pubic bone before, during and after passing water, are nearly always present. Sometimes there is a sensation of needing to urinate again just after the bladder has been emptied. The urine may be cloudy and smell quite unpleasant. The normal repeated doses of antibiotics are ineffective in most cases and eventually the organisms become resistant to antibiotics. But here again we have a golden opportunity for self-help. You must drink at least 3 pints of liquid each day. This should be mostly water. You must avoid all alcohol and coffee, but drink only very weak tea, or preferably herb teas. You should drink 4 glasses of barley water daily, made as follows. Boil 4 ounces of barley in half a pint of water for 5 minutes. Strain. Add one pint of cold water and the peel of half a lemon. Bring to the boil and simmer until the lemon is soft. Stand until cool, strain again and add 2 ounces of honey. You should eat a natural yoghurt each day. As with thrush, apply natural yoghurt to the vaginal and urethral openings morning and evening. Wear only cotton pants, wear stockings and not tights.

Women must always wipe their bottom from front to back, using a clean piece of paper for each wipe and not rubbing the paper backwards and forwards. Small girls should be taught to do this as early as possible. Women with cystitis or who get it frequently should try to pass urine as soon as possible after intercourse. Don't use coloured toilet paper – the dyes are sometimes irritant. Cut down on animal protein, citrus fruits, and avoid tomatoes, rhubarb, gooseberries, vinegar and pickles. You should take 500 mg of vitamin C each morning and each evening.

Both naturopathy and acupuncture can be helpful in the treatment of these distressing conditions and if you suffer recurrent bouts of either of them you should seek professional guidance.

Morning sickness

Morning sickness during the first three months of pregnancy affects 80 per cent of women. The feelings of nausea and actual vomiting most commonly occurring in the morning can happen at any time of the day or night. Even the smell of cooking, let alone eating food, can be enough to trigger off vomiting. In cases of severe and persistent vomiting it may be necessary for the mother to be hospitalised and for body fluids to be replaced with intravenous injections. To avoid damaging the growing baby, it is best to avoid all toxic medication unless absolutely essential.

Frequent small meals are usually better for the expectant mother suffering from morning sickness. A cup of tea with some dry toast or unsweetened wholemeal biscuits, preferably brought to the bedside first thing in the morning, will help to avoid the initial early morning nausea. Avoid fatty, greasy foods, coffee, strong tea and alcohol, and make sure that you eat plenty of good quality carbohydrates (you and the baby need the calories), wholemeal bread, wholewheat pasta, brown rice and plenty of fruit, salads and vegetables with fish or poultry and vegetarian sources as your main form of protein.

Provided the mother is in a good nutritional state before conception, the growing baby will get all the essential nutrients it needs from the mother's reserves. Early morning sickness will not in any way deprive the growing infant of nutrients.

Camomile tea last thing at night and first thing in the morning is a great help, although some women find that raspberry leaf tea or peppermint is preferable. Treatment with the homoeopathic remedies nux vomica or ipecacuanha also alleviates symptoms.

Fifty mg of vitamin B6 and 200 mg of magnesium taken each day together with a good multivitamin is also recommended.

Good food – better sex

Aphrodite was the Greek goddess of love and beauty, and it is from her name that we get the word 'aphrodisiac', which means a drug or food which excites sexual desire.

Our folk-lore is full of tales of these magic foods, but is there really any truth behind these old-wives', or perhaps they should be old-husbands', tales? Surprisingly, in spite of the fact that most people may scoff at the very notion of ordinary foods having any such power, there is some scientific evidence that many of the traditionally sexy foods may actually help.

First and foremost, it is essential to understand that nutrition is the vital factor. The body has an amazing ability to switch off sexual function when there is more important work for it to do. During and after any serious illness, it is unlikely that a woman will menstruate, or that a man will produce sperm. The same is true in cases of severe nutritional deprivation, anorexics soon stop having periods, as do many women athletes. In order to enjoy a normal, healthy and satisfying sex life, the prime need is for a good, varied and balanced diet.

Assuming that this is the case, what then of all the stories about food to boost your desires, or your partner's performance? There is no doubt about the romance of eating. A candle-lit dinner *à deux* is far more likely to end in consuming passion than fish and chips out of a newspaper on the kitchen table. Common sense should tell you that no man will be up to much after a meal of steak and kidney pud, spotted dick and bread and cheese, all washed down with several pints of his favourite brew.

A light meal of subtle flavours, foods that provide the essential vitamins and minerals, blend wonderful colours and won't overload the digestive system, is what is called for. Do go easy on the booze. A little wine, or better still champagne, will work wonders. But don't forget the infamous brewer's droop, or as Shakespeare warns more subtly in *Macbeth*: 'Drink . . . provokes the desire, but it takes away the performance.'

There are no magic foods or potions that will make up for a life of continual stress, that will compensate for a diet which does not provide enough protein, fats, carbohydrates, vitamins and minerals. On the other hand, there is no need for huge quantities of food – just look at the birth rates in some of the third world countries. In fact, the opposite is true. Obesity is a common cause of impotence and lack of sex drive. This may be purely the result of psychological problems, or physical changes connected with being overweight. Chronic back ache or arthritic hips do not make for good sexual performance.

There are many herbs which are reputed to have aphrodisiac properties. A mixture of rosemary and hibiscus is a simple favourite. Tea made of this combination certainly has a romantic and sensuous perfume. The ancient Greeks used the seeds of the ash tree which they claimed would 'render a man more spirited with the ladies'. The nasturtium, sometimes known as the 'flower of love', is not only delicious to eat, it cuts a romantic dash as a decoration on your dinner plate, and an infusion of the fresh leaves – half an ounce to a half-pint of boiling water – is thought to have a mild stimulating effect. In the Far East the powerful properties of ginseng are legendary, in fact its common name is 'man-root'.

One of the most famous of all sex books is the 16th-century *Perfumed Garden*. It advises men to eat strengthening foods like meat, eggs, aromatic herbs and sweetmeats made with honey.

From a scientific point of view the most important nutritional substances for normal sexual function are zinc; the B vitamins, B6 in particular; vitamins E, C and A; selenium and chromium.

Among the richest sources of zinc is the oyster, one of the most popular of all the supposed aphrodisiac foods. Casanova is said to have eaten at least fifty every day! Wheatgerm, oats, sesame and pumpkin seeds are also good sources of this vital substance. They are all rich in vitamin E as well, so it is hardly surprising that they too are part of the sex-food story.

Beef, liver, the humble herring and eggs are other good sources of these vitality-boosting ingredients, all of which crop up in the folk-lore of romance and love. There does seem to be a need for some animal protein in the diet. A man's interest in sex may be reduced on a totally vegetarian diet, though the same thing does not seem to happen to women. From my experience with patients, I think that it is the quality of diet which matters more. A bad meat eater and a bad vegetarian will suffer in just the same way. Anyone who lives on burger and beer, or white bread, pasta and puddings, is hardly going to make the world's most exciting lover. There is no doubt that a junk food diet high in the sweet and fatty foods will be low in those elements essential for all-round good health.

Asparagus, figs, bananas, leeks, caviar, mushrooms and even hot spices are regarded by some as aphrodisiacs. And remember that chocolate contains both caffeine and theobromine. The former is a stimulant and the latter a chemical that gives feelings of euphoria and happiness, just like being in love. Why do you think that all those ads for chocolate are romantic, adventurous or outright suggestive?

Some of these effects are chemical, some mere folk-lore, some the result of our own romantic expectations. It does not mater which, as if you believe in them they will work for you. What do not work, or if they do are extremely dangerous, are the patent medicines advertised as sexual stimulants. So save your money.

Intercourse is a simple physical act. Making love to a partner you care for is much more. The best aphrodisiac in the world is the touch or the cuddle of a loving, caring partner.

Or perhaps those three little words . . .

Curmonsky, chef to Napoleon, said: 'Properly speaking, there are no aphrodisiacs capable of endowing those blind to life with sight. But for those with poor eyesight in this matter, there are substances which act as magnifying lenses.'

Eating the right food will not miraculously cure all your sexual or reproductive problems. There are causes of infertility beyond the help of diet. There are problems of the reproductive system which will not respond to any magic foods. However, there are a huge range of conditions – some minor, and others more serious – for which the optimum eating plan can and will produce seemingly miraculous results.

Throughout history certain foodstuffs have been endowed with a near-magical influence on virility. Among them are sesame seeds, oysters, garlic, sarsparilla, liquorice, pollen and hops: the *Khama Sutra* specially recommended milk and honey! Research has shown that sesame seeds, oysters, garlic and milk – especially raw milk – are all excellent sources of zinc, without which active sperm cannot be formed; that sarsparilla, liquorice, pollen and hops all contain significant and easily available amounts of hormone-like substances; while honey, as well as supplying instant energy, contains minute amounts of many vital nutrients, and may also contain traces of pollen, which has been shown to have a beneficial action on the prostate gland.

Deprive animals of vitamin E and they become sterile, abort or miscarry. It's obviously impossible to carry out similar experiments with human beings, but all available evidence clearly shows that this vitamin is essential for successful reproduction.

Zinc deficiency is a common feature of many sexual problems, and the iron supplements almost routinely handed out to pregnant women only make matters worse by interfering with zinc uptake. Zinc deficiency is now known to be a factor in postnatal depression, premenstrual syndrome and menopausal women, and – together with folic acid – can easily be supplied to pregnant women by everyday foods in a form which does not cause bowel problems, nor interfere with mineral metabolism. Given the right tools for the job, your body can do a much better balancing act than your doctor can with synthetic supplements.

The enhanced need for zinc, iron and other minerals in sexual problems makes tea and coffee taboo, since they seriously impede mineral absorption. If you're desperate for the occasional cup of coffee or tea, make sure that you have it between meals.

Perhaps more than with any other health problem, the problems associated with the reproductive system demand the full rich spectrum of nutrition, with an extra measure of nutrients known to play a vital role – the B complex – particularly folic acid, vitamins A, C and E, the minerals iron, zinc and magnesium and plenty of good carbohydrates. This eating plan supplies them all.

Monday

Breakfast: Muesli, with extra sunflower, sesame and pumpkin seeds and orange juice.

Light meal or snack: Eggs mayonnaise with cayenne and toasted sesame seeds.

Main meal: Half a pink grapefruit. Liver casserole, potatoes and any green vegetable. Bananas with Greek yoghurt, sesame seeds and honey.

Tuesday

Breakfast: Scrambled eggs with tomatoes. Wholewheat toast, butter and honey.

Light meal or snack: Jacket potato with cottage cheese and chives. A dish of raisins, sultanas, pumpkin seeds and unsalted, fresh nuts.

Main meal: Raw mushrooms, in extra virgin olive oil, bay leaves, garlic, cider vinegar, rosemary and black pepper. A small grilled steak. Tomato and onion salad. Soaked dried fruits with a little cream and a few flaked almonds.

Wednesday

Breakfast: Porridge with cream and honey. Glass of orange juice to start with.

Light meal or snack: Sardines on wholemeal toast. Orange, pumpkin seeds and watercress salad. Rye crackers, cheese, grapes.

Main meal: Grilled chicken breasts, served with red lettuce and a salad of red, green and yellow peppers. Potatoes boiled in their skins. Fresh pineapple.

Thursday

Breakfast: Fresh fruit, Greek yoghurt with honey and nuts.

Light meal or snack: A selection of cheese with wholemeal roll and a beansprout salad. An apple.

Main meal: Chicken livers, fried in a little olive oil, sprinkled with black pepper and served on a bed of brown rice with a radish, rocket and fennel salad. A bunch of grapes.

Friday
Breakfast: An orange. Mushrooms on toast, large ones if you can get them, serve in their cooking juices, sprinkled with chopped parsley.
Light meal or snack: Salade Nicoise – hard boiled egg, tuna fish, cooked green beans, tomato, spring onion, cold boiled potato slices, lots of garlic and fresh chopped parsley. Crusty roll.
Main meal: Avocado, walnut and pear starter. Trout with almonds; mangetout peas, or broad beans, or broccoli. Sliced tomato and fresh basil salad. Baked apple filled with honey, sesame seeds, raisins and cinnamon.

Saturday
Breakfast: Orange and pineapple juice mixed. Two poached eggs on wholemeal toast.
Light meal or snack: A good vegetarian burger – I like 'Vegeburger' mixture the best. Beansprout salad with tomato, garlic, spring onion, parsley.
Main meal: Tsatsiki. Tandoori chicken with spiced rice, halva.

Sunday
Breakfast: Hot wholewheat rolls with butter and honey.
Light meal or snack: Cheese on toast, with mustard, and a green salad. Fresh fruit.
Main meal: for two. Celery and grape salad. Grilled salmon steaks with green sauce, with baby new potatoes boiled in their skins, and a tiny watercress salad – walnut oil and lemon dressing. A bowl of strawberries. A glass of good wine, soft music, candles – and no coffee.
'Coffee,' said Voltaire, 'is the beverage of eunuchs.'

Digestive disorders

Efficient functioning of the entire digestive system is an essential prerequisite to health. The dramatic and instant effects of brain damage, heart disease or kidney failure tend to overshadow the humble stomach. But it should never be forgotten that without proper breakdown of foods and the consequent availability to the entire system of vitamins, minerals, trace elements, micronutrients, fats, proteins and carbohydrates, all of which are vital to the very survival of every single cell in the body, the workings of these grander organs would come to a stop.

There are naturally serious and life-threatening disorders of the digestive system but, as a result of the highly dubious benefits of our Western society, the wide availability of convenience, processed, prepackaged and nutritionally deficient foodstuffs and the changing social patterns of the lifestyles that we all follow, millions of us are suffering from diseases of civilisation whose roots can be identified in the appalling way in which most of us treat our digestive systems.

Obesity, high blood pressure, heart disease, constipation, diverticular disease, appendicitis, piles, varicose veins, diarrhoea, headaches, cancer of the bowel, food allergies, hyperactivity in children, skin complaints, and many other conditions can all in part or totally be blamed on the way in which our diets have altered. Too much animal fat, too much sugar, too many artificial additives such as colourings, preservatives, flavourings, too little fibre, too little fresh fruit, vegetables, salads, too much meat, too much junk food: all these play a vital role in the general health of our nation. It takes mankind tens of thousands of years to make genetic changes in order to adapt to alterations in the environment. There have been more changes in our eating patterns in the last 100 years than in the previous 100,000, and we are not coping with them very well.

In 1977 American Senator George McGovern chaired an all-party report on the importance of diet to the American nation. McGovern's report said, 'The simple fact is that our diets have changed radically within the last 50 years with great and often very harmful effects on our health. Too much fat, too much sugar or salt can be and are linked directly to heart disease, cancer, obesity, stroke and other killer diseases. Those of us within government have an obligation to acknowledge this. The public wants guidance, wants to know the truth. In spite of all these factors the medical profession has still been slow to recognise the fundamental influence of nutrition on the general health, vitality and well-being of the population at large.'

These sentiments were echoed by our own National Advisory Committee on Nutrition Education, set up in Britain in 1979 (NACNE Report). The history of this report is a scandal. Dietary and nutritional experts, the Health Education Council, the Ministry of Agriculture, the food manufacturing industry – all were involved in the production of the report. The government did not like the findings and consequently the report was kept hidden and suppressed until finally it was leaked by *The Sunday Times* and in the *Lancet*, one of the most eminent of British medical journals. The official report was made public in September 1983 by the Health Education Council. The medical profession was agog. And finally the attitudes of the alternative health practitioners to nutrition were seen to be sound and sensible and not the rantings of the lunatic fringe. The NACNE Report produced a list of short-term goals which the British public should aim at in their dietary input:

(1) Reduce fat consumption by 10 per cent.
(2) Reduce sugar consumption by 10 per cent.
(3) Take more exercise.
(4) Increase fibre intake by 25 per cent.
(5) Reduce salt intake by 10 per cent.
(6) Reduce alcohol intake by 16 per cent.

Music to the ears of naturopaths like myself!

Many of the following problems are without doubt related to faulty nutrition. Often solutions are simple and lie firmly in your own hands, or rather your own mouth. One of the great pioneers of nature cure in this country was Stanley Lief, the founder of Champneys, and I heard him say on more than one occasion to a patient, 'You are digging your grave with your teeth'. The situation has not improved. The overall standards of nutrition have declined. Institutional catering in this country is a disgrace. The food served to our children in schools, to our sick people in hospitals, to our elderly in institutions, is doing more to encourage sickness and disease than any other single factor. Healthy eating is not a question of becoming a health freak or a vegetarian nut. It is a question of balance and common sense, and you will find many suggestions regarding nutrition and health in the Diet section at the back of the book (pages 261ff).

Colic

Most people associate colic with babies, who indeed get it very often. But adults can also suffer from this acutely painful condition. It is caused by muscle contractions in the digestive organs and it can result from conditions as diverse as constipation, colitis, gastro-enteritis, flatulence or diarrhoea.

In babies colic is often associated with food intolerance or allergy and studies have shown that cow's milk is a major factor in this distressing problem. Even breast-fed babies whose mothers consume large quantities of cow's milk have a much higher incidence of colic than those whose mothers do not consume cow's milk.

In both adults and babies isolated occurrences of colic, whilst uncomfortable, are no cause for alarm. But where there are repeated attacks of colic the underlying cause must be established, since merely alleviating the symptoms could cause further problems. The ever popular gripe water used for treating colic in babies is based on one of the traditional herbal remedies. Mix equal quantities of caraway, aniseed, and fennel seeds, and pound them to powder with a mortar and pestle. Add one teaspoon of this mixture to a cup of boiling water. Cover and allow to infuse for ten minutes. Strain and drink the water while it is still hot. For babies, one teaspoon of the water taken warm will provide effective relief.

Where the colic is obviously associated with flatulence, the use of charcoal tablets will provide dramatic relief, but again attention must be paid to any underlying dietary problems and the Hay system of eating is probably the most effective dietary regime for the treatment of recurrent and persistent flatulence. See Diet section at the back of the book (pages 261ff).

Colitis

This is an inflammatory condition of the lining of the lower part of the large bowel or colon, producing pain in the abdomen, diarrhoea, and frequently the passing of large quantities of mucus or even some blood mixed with the stool. Colitis is often associated with stress and anxiety conditions, and the attacks can be acute, or it can become a chronic disease. Infections of the colon or adverse reactions to some foods may be implicated.

Treatment with antibiotics or steroids or sometimes surgery to remove the damaged sections of the bowel may be required. No consideration of this problem can be complete without paying careful attention to the patient's diet. In many cases there are specific adverse reactions to some foods, particularly all dairy products and sometimes to meat and meat products.

It is important to keep a careful record of your total food intake over a period of several weeks, noting down when episodes of colitis occur. In this way it is possible to identify adverse reactions. These

169

foods can then be excluded from the diet. It may be worth trying a total exclusion diet, again keeping careful notes of what you eat, when you eat it and what reactions occur.

Acupressure to the points shown in the diagram will help to relieve the acute pain of intestinal spasm. You should add small quantities of fresh chickweed to your salad each day and take some slippery elm gruel morning and evening.

The homoeopathic remedies sulphur and arsenicum album are also useful. A daily dose of 500 mg of vitamin C, 25 mg of vitamin B6 and a high potency multivitamin pill should also be taken to ensure optimum vitamin levels.

As with most digestive disorders, the holistic approach is essential. A combination of a good diet, avoiding dairy products and including an adequate fibre intake is important, but this fibre should be obtained from brown rice, millet and buckwheat rather than ordinary wheat. A combination of therapies including naturopathy, acupuncture and relaxation therapies is ideal.

Constipation

Each year the British public spends £60 million on the purchase of the various laxative preparations which are available over the counter – £60 million which literally goes down the drain for no reason whatever other than faulty eating. The preponderance of refined flour products included in the British diet and the consequent lack of fibre is the major cause of constipation and all the ensuing problems related to this unnecessary and avoidable condition.

There are many misconceptions about constipation, but the key factor is the length of time which it takes for the digested food to pass through the large intestine. The longer that the faecal mass remains in the large bowel or colon, the more fluid is absorbed from it and the harder this mass becomes, resulting in compacted hardened stools which become difficult to pass. In practice I have found that many patients who suffer from this uncomfortable disorder not only consume too little fibre, but also drink far too little liquid, the ideal minimum being a fluid intake of 3 pints daily.

The frequency of bowel movement is not the key indicator in constipation. Rather it is the quality of the stool passed and ideally this should be soft and formless, but not of course watery. Varicose veins and piles are two of the commonest side effects of constipation and these are caused by the enormous strain and effort required to pass a hard stool. Whilst it is true that most cases of constipation are self-inflicted, there are some commonly prescribed drugs, particularly painkillers, iron tablets and antidepressants which can cause constipation, and there is no doubt that anxiety, stress and tension, and obsessional attitudes to bowel function also play an important role.

The long-term use of laxatives, especially those of the purgative type, is definitely not a good idea. These chemicals are irritant to the bowel and can firstly produce dependence on them, and secondly cause damage to the sensitive membranes which line the large intestine.

Many people may suffer the odd occurrence of constipation which can be easily treated with simple natural laxatives. Syrup of figs, dried apricots, prunes and extra fibre, together with an increased fluid intake, will all help. However, if you have normally had a perfectly adequate bowel function and suddenly start getting constipated, particularly if this constipation alternates with bouts of diarrhoea, you should seek medical help urgently. The cause may be quite simply a change in dietary habits, stress or medication, but it may be an indicator of some obstructive bowel disease which should be investigated.

For the majority of people, the simple expedient of increasing the amount of cereal fibre that you eat to about 30 g per day, and making sure that you drink adequate liquids, is all that is normally required. There are various proprietary preparations on the market which contain bran, but continuing with your poor dietary habits and just taking a few tablets is not the real answer. Increase the amount of wholemeal bread that you eat, increase your intake of other wholemeal cereals, brown rice, wholemeal pasta, all the bean family, and don't forget the vegetable fibre which you get from fruits, salads and vegetables. Although this is beneficial, it is not a substitute for cereal fibre. The simple addition of a couple of dessertspoons of bran to your morning cereal or stirred into your yoghurt will normally suffice. Be careful not to take excessive quantities of bran, however, as this can combine with other minerals, particularly calcium, and make them more difficult for the body to absorb. Porridge is one of the best forms of fibre.

Acupressure applied to the points on the diagram will certainly help, as will herbal treatment with one tablespoon of linseeds soaked overnight in water and added to your breakfast cereal. Tea made from an infusion of sennapods is also beneficial in the treatment of stubborn constipation.

Rhythmic massage of the abdomen following the line of the colon can also help to start the normal wavelike contractions of the colon wall. This should be done in a clockwise direction, starting at the bottom right-hand corner of the abdomen and ending in the bottom left-hand corner.

Ten mg of vitamin B1 and a B complex taken daily will also help, especially taken in conjunction with a carton of natural yoghurt every morning. Psychotherapy and relaxation techniques can help to overcome underlying problems of stress or bowel obsession while professional manipulative treatment from an osteopath and acupuncture can also be employed if self-help fails.

Diarrhoea

Acute bouts of diarrhoea may be the result of excessive anxiety, for example, just before an important interview or examination; or after eating large quantities of laxative foods, prunes, figs, plums, or underripe fruits. However, the most important cause of diarrhoea is infection. Bacteria and viruses may both cause diarrhoea and this can also be associated with vomiting.

Poor hygiene and ineffective water purification are the key factors in this problem. Over 60 per cent of people who travel abroad return having had some form of stomach upset. Once you set foot outside Britain, Northern Europe or North America, you are at risk. Standards of hygiene, especially in parts of the Mediterranean, India and Africa, can be appallingly low. Do not be fooled into a false sense of security by staying at luxury hotels, since most gastric bugs are distributed by flies and they can't read the price list! In these countries avoid drinking the water, and do not put ice cubes in your drink. Stick to branded drinks in sealed containers and make sure they come to your table still sealed. Do not eat salads or any fruit which you cannot peel. Never eat undercooked meat or fish and avoid the now ubiquitous cold buffet. Cold meats or a dish of mayonnaise standing in the hot Mediterranean sun is a haven for all sorts of bacteria. Before eating in a restaurant, look at the toilet: if there are flies there, there are certainly flies in the kitchen – go somewhere else. More often you are better off eating simple local foods rather than trying the more expensive smart restaurants. After all, today's lunch may simply be last night's dinner rearranged. Sardines grilled over glowing charcoal, or a kebab cooked on the hot coals before your eyes, is often a better bet and less likely to cause problems. Avoid ice cream, another haven for bacteria.

Diarrhoea can be brought on by some drugs, particularly antibiotics, and it is sound practice to make sure that you always take natural yoghurt and a vitamin B complex tablet whenever you are prescribed a course of antibiotics, and that you continue with this regime for at least ten days after you have finished the medicine.

For whatever reason, diarrhoea can be most serious in the very young and the very old. The drastic fluid loss which occurs can cause dehydration and a serious imbalance between the body's minerals, particularly sodium and potassium. Any bout of acute diarrhoea and vomiting which has not resolved itself within 24 to 48 hours should be referred immediately for professional examination. In the meantime, the essential is to maintain the patient's fluid intake and with small children this is best done by giving them a dessertspoon of liquid every 10 to 15 minutes. This should not be ice-cold but tepid water, diluted fruit juices, any sort of fluid, but not milk. In some cases it may be advisable to add a little sugar and a pinch of salt to the fluid.

When babies get recurrent episodes of colic and diarrhoea, this may be a sign of food intolerance. The most common food causing these problems is likely to be cow's milk and all milk products. These should be avoided, and even if the baby is being breast-fed a high intake of cow's milk by the mother can adversely affect the baby, so she too should cut down on her cow's milk intake.

Garlic tablets will help, especially if taken at night. During the first 24 hours of a bout of diarrhoea avoid all food, then gradually introduce liquidised soups, vegetable juices, yoghurt, and then feed boiled rice, steamed carrots, bananas, dry toast, and gradually go back to normal. A good mineral supplement, particularly including sodium and potassium, is essential to replace what has been lost during the attack.

Remember, in small babies and elderly people, diarrhoea can be extremely serious. Don't delay, seek professional advice immediately.

The use of proprietary medicines to stop attacks of diarrhoea is not advisable except in emergency situations (trains, travelling etc.). If there is a serious cause like food poisoning, you may mask the symptoms before getting proper treatment.

Diverticulitis

This is another of the diseases of our Western civilised diet. The absence of cereal fibre causes constipation and the effort required to push the resulting hard dry stools through the colon creates a dramatic rise in pressure in this organ. This pressure causes small pockets or diverticula to bulge out of the wall of the colon. Faecal material gets trapped in these pockets and causes infection. This can lead to severe pain, bleeding, mucus, diarrhoea, nausea and even vomiting.

Until just a few years ago the standard medical treatment for this condition was a prescription of a totally bland diet. Conversely the naturopaths have always advocated an increase of fibre. This bone of contention between orthodox and unorthodox medicine was finally resolved by Dr Denis Burkitt, a world-renowned medical specialist. He observed whilst working in Africa that the native African who lived on his traditional diet never suffered from diverticular disease, appendicitis, colitis, or even cancer of the bowel, and yet when these Africans changed to the Western way of eating they suffered these illnesses in the same proportion as the Europeans. As a result of Burkitt's observations, the entire medical profession has gradually switched to naturopathic methods of treating this disease. The success has been phenomenal. A condition which was frequently treated by surgical removal of the affected part of the bowel is now nearly always totally resolved by the simple expedient of adding bran to the diet.

Sadly, as with many alternative practices, the doctors ignore the underlying philosophies and use the treatment on a purely symptomatic basis. Hence patients are often prescribed fibre tablets for the treatment of the condition. Whilst it is undoubtedly true that this is a very quick way of removing the patient from a consulting room, it does nothing to re-educate and reform eating habits. It does nothing to change the dietary patterns of families, and consequently perpetuates the illness which could, if the British public changed their diets tomorrow, be a thing of the past in twenty years' time.

As in the treatment of constipation, an increase in fluid and cereal fibre in the diet is the first step. Chamomile tea taken before meals, and the use of slippery elm gruel twice daily during acute attacks, will also bring some dramatic relief. For many sufferers it is important to reduce the amount of dairy products eaten and also to avoid red meat, coffee, alcohol and all refined carbohydrate products. A mixture of carrot, apple and celery juice is healing to the lining of the colon and regular dosing with high-potency slow-release vitamin B complex helps to encourage formation of the natural bacteria whose presence is so vital to the functioning of the digestive system.

Naturopathy, acupuncture, manipulative treatment to stimulate the nerve supply to the digestive organs, and frequently the use of relaxation therapies, will all help to overcome this distressing but nearly always curable illness.

Flatulence

The embarrassment of wind affects us all at some time or another. Whether simply the result of swallowing too much air when eating or drinking, eating large quantities of foods which produce excessive gases, like the bean family, or whether caused by some underlying disease like diverticulitis, ulcers, irritable bowel syndrome, or even hiatus hernia, the condition is uncomfortable, and can become a social disadvantage. Most commonly, bad eating habits are the sole cause and these are easily remedied. Avoiding food combinations likely to produce more gas is the first step. See the Hay dietary system at the back of the book (page 272). For the relief of isolated occurrences, charcoal biscuits or tablets are extremely effective, but as with all symptomatic treatments, not a substitute for curing the root cause of the problem. If you have recently increased the amount of fibre in your diet you can expect to experience a certain amount of wind until your digestive system has adapted to these changes. Make sure that you eat slowly, chewing your food thoroughly, and keeping your mouth closed. Too much talking and eating at the same time is a sure way of increasing the problem.

Peppermint tea after meals and the addition of sage, rosemary and thyme to your cooking will also help.

It is certain that people under excessive stress and those of a highly nervous and anxious disposition are more likely to suffer from this problem. Psychotherapy and relaxation techniques are of immense benefit, but the first step is to consult a naturopath for advice on your eating patterns.

Gall-stones

Fair, fat, fertile, forty, female and flatulent. This is the person most likely to get gall-stones. Up to 10 per cent of the population will have them, and five times as many women as men. Yet again, a disease of civilisation related to high fat intakes and obesity.

The gall-bladder stores bile, which is produced by the liver and essential for the breakdown of fats. The bile is passed through a small duct into the digestive system and, when the stones obstruct this duct, a sequence of most unpleasant symptoms arises. Called biliary colic, it starts as an extremely severe pain in the abdomen, which moves across to the right. Accompanied by nausea and severe vomiting, the pain can last for hours and frequently causes referred pain to the right side and the right shoulder blade. Due to the blockage of the bile duct, jaundice frequently occurs after an acute attack of biliary colic. Normally the gall-bladder is removed, but it is always worth trying complete dietary change before undergoing this operation unless the attacks are so severe and frequent as to disrupt normal life totally.

The first step is to remove all fats from the diet: red meat, sausages, salamis, pâtés, bacon, ham, meat pies, corned beef – in fact all meat products, together with all dairy products, cheeses, creams, ice creams, cakes, biscuits, any of which are likely to contain considerable amounts of saturated fats. The diet should contain a high proportion of raw vegetables, raw fruits, raw salads, and plenty of cereal fibre, especially wholemeal bread, wholemeal pasta and brown rice. Take particular care to include dandelion leaves and globe artichokes regularly, since these have a beneficial effect on the gall-bladder itself. Poultry should be eaten without the skin, and plenty of fish. Avoid all fried foods and eggs.

A dessertspoonful of safflower seed oil, 500 mg of vitamin C and 400 iu of vitamin E would all help to reduce the cholesterol content of the bile.

Since the majority of sufferers are likely to be women, it is essential to maintain adequate calcium intake, particularly approaching the time of the menopause. For this reason, since you will be cutting out nearly all dairy products (you may be able to introduce low fat yoghurts and cheeses as your condition improves), you must make sure that you take an adequate calcium and vitamin D supplement on a daily basis, Porosis D is the best.

Although all these self-help measures make a considerable difference, it is important that you get professional advice and the most useful forms of complementary therapy for the treatment of gall-stones are naturopathy, acupuncture and homoeopathy.

Gastroenteritis

(See Diarrhoea, page 172.) Nausea, vomiting, and diarrhoea combined with severe abdominal cramp is almost certain to be gastroenteritis. Caused by an inhaled virus which spreads extremely rapidly in an enclosed community like a school, hospital or old people's home, it can be extremely serious in small children and the elderly. Sometimes the condition is caused by bacteria – particularly salmonella linked with food poisoning, and inevitably the result of poor food hygiene, wrong handling and storage of foods or an infected carrier working with food.

In babies the commonest cause of gastroenteritis is poor sterilisation and hygiene when the baby is being bottle fed. The treatment is identical to that for diarrhoea.

Any small child with constant vomiting and diarrhoea should be seen by a medical practitioner, unless the symptoms show signs of resolving within six hours.

Gingivitis

Most people commonly lose their teeth through gum disease rather than tooth disease, and gingivitis is the commonest of these. More than three-quarters of the population will suffer from gingivitis at some time during their lives, nearly always because they don't pay sufficient care to the way in which they look after their teeth or mouth. This problem is also common in alcoholics or may be the result of some long-standing illness or lack of vitamin C in the diet.

The first sign of gingivitis is that your gums bleed very easily. Brushing the teeth or even eating an apple can be sufficient to start them off. Swelling and inflammation are always present and, if left untreated, the gums and surrounding bone can become severely damaged. Pus can collect around the bottom of the teeth and may cause tooth abscesses. Bad breath is an inevitable consequence.

Poor diet and poor dental hygiene increase the possibility of gingivitis occurring. A lack of raw fruit, vegetables or salads, together with an over-indulgence in highly refined carbohydrates, sticky sweets, sweetened drinks, all create the right environment for bacteria to multiply and for plaque to develop on the teeth and minimise the massaging effect that chewing fibrous foods has on the gums.

Teeth must be brushed whenever possible after eating, but certainly not less than morning and bedtime. The use of dental floss also helps to prevent the build-up of plaque.

Many years ago a dentist gave me a recipe for a mouthwash which was given to him by his father, also a dentist. This prescription is useful for any form of mouth or gum infection, but particularly in the treatment of gingivitis.

Add two teaspoons of 20 volume hydrogen peroxide to a tumbler full of warm water. Rinse the mouth thoroughly, using the whole glassful, forcing the water between your teeth and swilling around the mouth. Spit out – do not swallow. Now add one teaspoon of Milton to half a glass of hot water and repeat the same rinsing action. Again, do not swallow. Although the Milton tastes awful, do not rinse your mouth out immediately afterwards. This procedure should be repeated every time you eat, where practical, but certainly after breakfast and last thing at night.

Regular treatment with 7500 iu of vitamin A and 200 iu of vitamin E taken daily and the homoeopathic remedy mercurius solubilis will also help.

If you have recurring problems with bleeding gums, do see your dentist without delay. It could save your teeth.

Irritable bowel syndrome (IBS)

Severe abdominal pain, distention, diarrhoea, or alternating constipation and diarrhoea, are typical of this distressing problem. IBS may happen after gastroenteritis or repeated courses of antibiotics. There are often changes in the natural bacteria in the intestines, although all normal routine investigations seldom show any specific problems. For this reason many doctors believe that IBS is purely a psychological problem, which for the vast majority of patients is absolutely not true. Naturally, weeks, months or even years of severe pain and discomfort are enough to depress anyone, but the depression is the result of the problem, not the other way round.

For many years naturopaths have treated IBS as some form of adverse food reaction or food allergy, a belief which has been justified by recent research work at Cambridge: 182 patients with IBS were treated by Hunter, Jones and Workman, by changing their diets; 122 patients were completely relieved of their symptoms and two years later, 71 were contacted again. Of these, 59 were still following the diet and well, and 6 of them had gone back to normal eating and had not suffered any form of relapse. The only treatment was the use of exclusion diets to identify the irritant foods and then advising the patients to remain on the food regime which had been found most suitable for them.

Dairy products, red meats and wheat products were found to be the most frequent irritants and, as any naturopath would have suggested years before, increasing the natural fibre content of the diet, reducing the amount of meat and animal fats, and reducing the refined carbohydrates is the answer for most people suffering from this condition. How much better than the inevitable prescription of tranquillisers which can affect the muscles of the intestines, making it even more probable that the sufferers will also have to contend with diarrhoea.

As with all ongoing bowel problems, it is important to ensure adequate vitamin and mineral intakes, therefore a good quality high-potency multivitamin and mineral supplement should be taken. Whilst acupuncture treatment will help to relieve the worst of the symptoms of this condition, ideally it should be treated by a naturopath and consideration given to the overall dietary changes required for each individual.

Liver problems

Serious problems affecting the liver have the most dire medical consequences. Hepatitis, alcohol abuse, drug toxicity, cancer and parasites can all create life-threatening situations which are outside the scope of self-help or alternative therapy.

However, general malaise and 'liverishness' frequently affect overall well-being and can be tackled with simple but effective alternative means.

An over-indulgence in alcohol, rich fatty foods, and a generally poor nutritional intake will all have adverse effects on the liver. Acupressure of the points illustrated will bring considerable relief, although for ongoing liver problems the advice of an acupuncturist should be sought.

Rosemary, peppermint or camomile teas provide gentle stimulation to liver function and the homoeopathic remedy bryonia is always useful.

A few weeks on a totally fat-free naturopathic diet with fruit and plenty of raw vegetables will also provide rapid relief from minor liver complaints. Celery juice and extract of artichoke should be

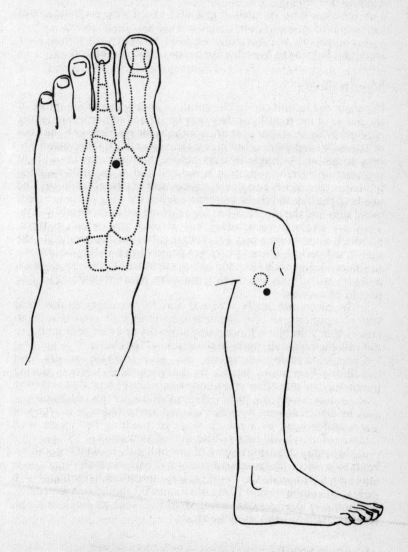

Acupressure points for the relief of 'liverishness'. For
acupressure instructions, see caption on page 94

taken regularly. Plenty of still mineral water, a gentle massage over the liver region and the application of cold packs to the abdomen will also be beneficial.

A tablespoonful of lecithin granules taken with each meal and high doses of vitamin C up to 3 g daily should also be taken.

A naturopath will certainly be able to help with minor liver ailments, but severe liver disease needs medical attention.

Mouth ulcers

Ulcers in the mouth can be the result of injury, especially biting of the inside of the mouth, or they may be related to herpes, but most commonly some 80 per cent are aphthous ulcers. Between the ages of 10 and 40 and more often in females than males, these ulcers are very common. A couple of days before the ulcer appears a slight soreness or burning sensation is noticed and as the inflammation increases, the ulcers become apparent and extremely painful. The inside of the lips and cheeks and the edge of the tongue are the most usual sites and the ulcer can last for anything between 4 and 14 days. They are likely to recur often but without any regular pattern, although some women may get them regularly just at the start of the menstrual period. Once you've got some ulcers, eating becomes a problem. Acidic foods like tomatoes, citrus fruits, vinegar, pickles, and very spicy foods like curries, make the pain excruciating. These should be avoided.

If the ulcers are really severe it may be necessary to use local steroid applications, but the first step is to visit your dentist to ensure that your bite is functioning normally and that your teeth are not causing repeated injury to the inside of the cheek.

Chronic digestive disorders can also increase acidity and conditions like hiatus hernia or early morning sickness during pregnancy, or any other condition which causes repeated vomiting (see Anorexia nervosa, page 183), can all trigger this condition.

A herbal treatment with half a teaspoon of red sage in a cup of warm water used as a mouth wash or painting the ulcers with tincture of myrrh will help reduce the inflammation.

A three-day cleansing regime of raw or lightly cooked vegetables, vegetable juices and non-acid fruits and excluding all other foods may help to eliminate the ulcers rapidly, and vitamin treatment with 7500 iu of vitamin A and 10 mg of vitamin B2 should be taken daily. Sucking zinc lozenges containing vitamin C such as ZinCold is also an effective way to shorten the attack.

Stomach ache

Overindulgence is the most likely cause of stomach ache. Rich food, drink, too much fat, or even just too much, can cause pain in the stomach. Even the wrong combinations of foods can cause discomfort, and so long as there is no sudden weight loss, continual pain, loss of blood with the stool, or repeated bouts of diarrhoea or vomiting, all of which could be indicative of underlying disease, then the occasional bout of stomach ache is an uncomfortable though minor irritation.

Stress, tension and anxiety may be the cause, but here again the odd isolated episode is no reason for alarm. Acupressure on the points of the diagram will help relieve the pain fairly quickly and peppermint tea is an effective specific remedy.

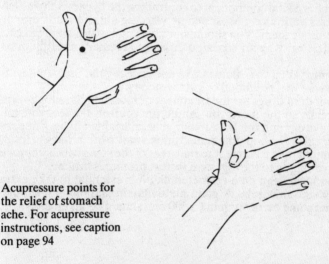

Acupressure points for the relief of stomach ache. For acupressure instructions, see caption on page 94

For children with stomach ache, mix one teaspoon of powdered slippery elm bark with some honey and dissolve in a cup of boiling water. Allow to cool and let the child sip. This can be repeated up to three times daily.

Reducing the caffeine intake and the amount of fats in the diet, and cutting down on smoking – preferably stop altogether – will all help to minimise recurrent episodes of stomach ache. Where stress is involved, then learning some form of relaxation therapy is a great help.

Ulcers

Duodenal ulcers occur in the lining of the duodenum and they can be caused by excessive acidity or enzyme action. There is no doubt that stress is a key factor in these ulcers. Gastric ulcers are found in the stomach, but they are less frequent than duodenal ulcers and occur mostly in older men.

These type of ulcers are not suitable for self-treatment and professional help is essential, but there are a number of pointers which will help you to recover more quickly. Don't smoke, don't abuse alcohol (a little is OK). Bland diets, so often recommended, are not the answer, since they can lead to vitamin and mineral deficiencies and cause other bowel problems. Introduce cereal and vegetable fibres gradually. You can take your vegetables as liquidised soups or purées.

You must learn to relax properly and some form of relaxation technique is a vital component to controlling the hyperacidity which aggravates your ulcer. Most people who use antacid medicines or tablets misuse them. You should not take them with a meal but two hours afterwards, with repeated doses as necessary until the next meal.

You must keep your fluid intake up, since regular use of antacids can increase the likelihood of kidney stones.

The modern drugs for the treatment of ulcers do have long-term side effects, so the more you can do for yourself the less you will need the drugs and the better your general health will be. Slippery elm and the homoeopathic remedy nux vomica are always helpful, and manipulative treatment to the areas of the spine which improve the nerve supply to the digestive system promotes healing.

If you have been on a restricted diet it is essential to take extra vitamins and minerals. A good multivitamin and mineral supplement and some extra vitamin C, 500 mg, should be taken daily.

Problems of the nervous system

Anorexia nervosa and Bulimia nervosa

The word anorexia means nothing more than loss of appetite. It can arise following diseases involving the mouth and teeth, the digestive system, acute infections, exhaustion or even sometimes as the result of some forms of drug treatment.

Anorexia nervosa is a very different, serious and sometimes even life-threatening illness which develops as a result of deep-seated anxiety neurosis. Those suffering with this wretched problem refuse to eat sufficient food to maintain their bodily functions. They are not even able to admit that they need additional food. Frequently food becomes repellent. As a result of family pressures, the anorexic devises all kind of tricks to cover up the illness: hiding their food, chewing it and spitting it out when no one is looking, finding endless excuses for not being at home when the rest of the family sit down to eat a meal, or often just plain lying. When placed in a situation where they cannot avoid eating, they will make themselves sick at the earliest opportunity or swallow huge doses of laxative medicines. I had one patient whose friend discovered forty empty laxative wrappers in just one day hidden around the house.

A study at Great Ormond Street Hospital for Children showed that, contrary to popular belief, more and more boys are suffering from this dreadful condition. In fact, up to 25 per cent of the patients referred to the hospital with anorexia were boys.

Anorexia is the physical manifestation of deep-seated emotional disturbances nearly always arising out of difficulties in the patient's interpersonal relationships, mostly with their families and especially with their own mother. Patients are frequently thin to the point of emaciation, although at the same time obsessed with their own image of themselves as being fat. Since this condition prevents the onset of menstruation or stops it from occurring, it is sometimes believed that young girls particularly are trying to avoid growing up. There may have been some particular emotional disturbance such as the death of a parent, the loss of a brother or sister, or divorce, or there may be a long history of stormy relationships within the family, but whatever the causes, treatment is extremely difficult and often unsuccessful. Severe cases will need hospitalisation and both medical and psychiatric treatment. Complementary therapies can be used, but in conjunction with orthodox treatment. Healing and hypnosis are effective. Nutritional counselling and psychotherapy are vital and in this context I have seen the best results where the family receives therapy as a group as well as individual treatment for the patient. Learning relaxation techniques such as yoga and meditation will help the sufferer to cope more easily with the stresses of their daily life.

Zinc deficiency is common in anorexics and high doses of up to 150 mg daily should be taken initially and, as the patient starts to improve, this can be reduced to a regular dose of 15 mg three times a day.

Bulimia nervosa is a similar illness which involves abnormal eating patterns. In this situation the patient is likely to swing from huge eating binges to virtual starvation. After bingeing, they usually induce vomiting or take enormous doses of laxatives.

The bulimic patient is normally considerably older than the anorexic, the disease being most common in the middle twenties.

Bulimics are normally able to camouflage their condition far more satisfactorily since, when they are in a social situation, they appear to be eating normally and they are seldom as emaciated as the anorexic. The root causes are much the same and the treatments similar. Psychotherapy, nutritional rehabilitation and counselling, and a determined effort to prevent the habitual use of laxatives, are vital, since long-term use of these types of drugs can cause serious damage to the digestive system.

Apart from the obvious cause of anorexic disease, the long-term outlook, even for those who recover, can sometimes be rather bleak. Sterility, bowel disorders and inflammation caused by constant vomiting can all produce long-term effects which may take years to clear.

Anxiety

Every one of us has experienced anxiety – the pounding of the heart when frightened, the feeling of excitement, the urgent need to pass water at times of great stress – but someone with anxiety neurosis experiences these fears and anxieties with an intensity that bears little or no relation to the true situation.

There is a tendency for anxiety neurosis to run in families, but the most likely cause is usually to be found in episodes which occur in childhood. Rapid heart-rate, perspiring, and acute feelings of tension accompany the idea that some dreadful event is constantly imminent. Occasionally this type of neurosis can develop into a phobia: a fear of electricity, a fear of flying, a fear of leaving the house, a fear of being alone or a fear of being with other people. At its worst a sense of real panic develops and the sufferer can feel totally overwhelmed by terror.

Hypochondria is a common bedfellow to anxiety neurosis. There are frequently morbid obsessions with bodily functions and disease. It is important that these physical symptoms should be investigated. The negative results can help to allay the fears of the patient and in any case it must never be forgotten that even hypochondriacs do get ill. Loss of appetite, insomnia, hyperventilation, hyperactivity, bad temper and copious sweating, especially on the palms and on the forehead, all are signs of this condition. The patient may appear confused, and even making the simplest decisions can be extremely difficult.

This disorder is usually treated with drugs, especially tranquillisers, but antidepressants and sleeping pills are also often prescribed. Used in isolation these drugs do nothing to help the patient overcome this disabling illness. Counselling is the first step and your counsellor may be a trained professional, a priest, a friend or even your next-door neighbour, but a sympathetic ear is often a great healer. Acupressure treatment can help to diminish the most acute symptoms and should be applied to the points shown on the

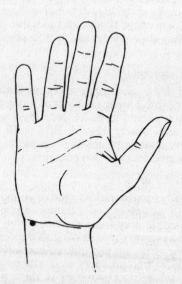

Acupressure points for the reief of anxiety and
insomnia. For acupressure instructions, see caption
on page 94

diagram. Herbal treatment with Bio-Strath valerian formula, a mixture of valerian and passiflora extracts, is extremely useful as a gentle calmative. The homoeopathic remedy aconite or lycopodium is also helpful. There is no doubt that regular massage and manipulative treatment to relieve the secondary muscle tension which can in itself become a cause of the problem should also be used, but a combination of sound nutrition, regular exercise and psychotherapy are the real answers to this difficulty. Learning to come to terms with your emotional problems and using anger and aggression in a positive manner, especially when combined with an improvement in family situations and self-esteem, will all help towards a deeper understanding and a better coping mechanism.

High potency B complex taken morning and evening together with 200 mg of vitamin C three times daily should also be added to the regime.

Depression

Every one of us experiences depression at some time in our lives, normally as a result of such distressing events as bereavement, divorce, loss of job, failure to succeed in some enterprise. There are, however, those for whom depressive illness becomes a major problem. Broadly speaking, depressive illness can be divided into endogenous depressive illness and reactive depression. These are two very different problems and it is important to understand the differences.

Endogenous depression

This form of depression seems to occur with no apparent reason. The sufferers exhibit feelings of loss of self-esteem, guilt and doubt. They are often unable to make even the simplest of decisions for themselves and nearly always they suffer from severe sleep disorders. Physical symptoms like headaches, anorexia and general digestive disturbances are also common.

Reactive depression

This is normally seen in middle aged or younger people and appears together with symptoms of extreme anxiety. In the depths of depression people may frequently contemplate and even achieve suicide, which is a very real risk for all depressive patients. The use of anti-depressant drugs and electro-convulsive therapy sometimes combined with tranquillisers and sleeping pills does little to alleviate the underlying problems in these patients. Drug therapy may well be the only treatment when depressives are in extremis, but this should always be looked upon as a short-term measure used to get the patient through a particular crisis. Sadly, all too often the drugs are administered on long-term repeat prescriptions with very little assessment of the patient's progress.

The National Association for Mental Health, MIND, recently produced a report on anti-depressant drugs which made very depressing reading. Each year, they say, some 400 people commit suicide by taking an overdose of anti-depressant drugs. Seven-and-a-half million prescriptions for these drugs are written by doctors each year and over a twenty-year period three-quarters of all women and more than half of all men will visit their doctor with a mental health problem, and most of the women and many of the men will have at least one episode of depression.

Whilst anti-depressants can be very effective, they do have side effects, some of which are serious, and most doctors don't give their patients enough information about these drugs in order for them to make informed decisions as to whether or not they want to take them.

Counselling, psychotherapy and support from family and friends are often all that's needed; after all, some 60 per cent of people suffering from depression get better without any treatment whatsoever.

Writing a prescription is the easiest way for the doctor to end the consultation and now that most people know about the dangers of the massive over-prescription of tranquillisers during the last thirty years, MIND is concerned that doctors will simply prescribe other potentially more dangerous drugs like anti-depressants. Don't let the doctor fob you off with a prescription for these powerful medicines – it may solve his or her problem but it won't necessarily solve yours.

Insist that your doctor explains what he is prescribing, what it's called, what it's for, what side effects it may have and exactly how you should take it, particularly whether or not it is necessary to avoid eating certain foods in conjunction with the drug. This is important since the anti-depressant drugs which are monoamine-oxidase inhibitors can react badly with some foods and cause very toxic side effects. If you are prescribed these drugs, you should absolutely avoid all cheese, oxo, bovril, marmite or similar meat and yeast extracts, broad bean pods, pickled herrings, bananas, yoghurt, chocolate, canned figs, most red wines and sherry, although all alcohol should be drunk in moderation or best avoided. The common proprietary names for these MAOAIs are Nardil, Marsilid, Marplan and Parnate.

Above all, remember that anti-depressant drugs should be the last resort and not the first choice in the treatment of depressive illness.

Whilst some of the herbal remedies like hops, passiflora, valerian or lavender may be helpful, and the homoeopathic remedies of Nat.

Mur., arsenicum album may help, psychotherapy is the form of treatment most likely to succeed. Improving self-awareness, group therapy, counselling and encouraging the depressive to talk about his or her problems is the first step on the road to recovery.

Relaxation techniques, hypnosis and massage to encourage relaxation can also be tried successfully. Regular doses of 50 mg of vitamin B6, a good multivitamin preparation and 200 mg of magnesium should be taken for at least three months.

Dizziness

Dizziness is a sensation of movement of the surroundings or the sensation of things 'spinning round' inside the head. The sensation can be one of rotating or a feeling of displacement in just one direction. There is nearly always an accompanying problem of balance and the patient looks for something to lean on. In sudden and severe attacks falls may occur and the sufferer is likely to break out into a cold sweat, feel sick, look pale and sometimes even faint. True vertigo may be caused by lesions in the brain, but it is also a common problem in people suffering from anxiety neuroses. Ear diseases may also cause problems of balance, particularly Ménière's Disease or infections of the balance mechanism or even damage caused by some diseases like mumps or some drugs like quinine, aspirin or streptomycin.

Arthritic changes in the small bones of the neck can also cause a restriction of the blood supply by kinking the arteries that lead to the brain and this in turn may cause dizziness.

Postural hypotension, that is a sudden drop in blood pressure when you move quickly from a lying to a sitting position or from sitting to standing, may cause a momentary fall in blood pressure leading to transient giddiness.

Chronic sinus infections or persistent catarrh may also cause obstruction in the Eustachian tube with consequent changes of the pressure inside the ear.

It is essential that an accurate diagnosis as to the cause of dizziness be arrived at. In most cases the causes are not serious, but just occasionally there may be underlying conditions requiring medical intervention.

Acupuncture can be useful in relieving this problem and self-help with the pressure points illustrated can bring rapid relief. Homoeopathic treatment with gelsemium or pulsatilla and massage to the sinuses, head and neck can all be beneficial. If chronic catarrh is the underlying problem, then changes in diet are nearly always helpful. As with most catarrhal problems, the first thing to try is removing all dairy products from the food intake. Homoeopathic treatment is essential where arthritis of the neck is interfering with

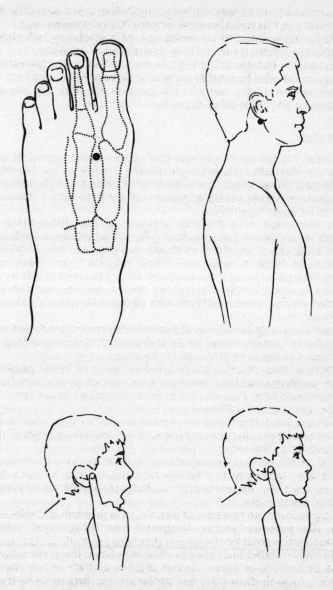

Acupressure points for the relief of dizziness. For
acupressure instructions, see caption on page 94

the normal blood supply, although this should not normally be undertaken in this situation without prior X-ray examinations.

Where the problem is obviously one of a psychological origin, and this is particularly true where patients have a constant fear of falling, psychotherapy is the key to success. The use of relaxation therapies and even hypnotherapy may achieve good results.

Regular doses of a megadose vitamin B complex are recommended for all problems of dizziness.

Migraine

There can't be many people who don't either suffer from or know someone who suffers from this distressing condition. The blinding headaches, the sickness, the sensitivity to noise and light and the wretchedness of the severe migraine sufferer have only to be seen once to be never forgotten.

It's important to distinguish between people suffering from tension headaches and those suffering from true migraine. Even the worst headache bears no resemblance to a migraine attack. I have seen many patients who have been told or have diagnosed themselves as suffering from migraine simply because this is more socially acceptable than describing their condition as a stress reaction. We are concerned here with the miseries of unmistakable migraine.

The causes of this condition are complex and may include adverse reactions to certain foods, stress and anxiety, hormone changes, high blood pressure or problems in the neck area of the spine.

Whilst women are more likely to suffer than men, in children the illness is divided equally amongst boys and girls, and although migraine usually begins after puberty, it can happen at any time.

Migraines occur in different ways in different people. Some suffer the weekend migraine: after they have coped with the stresses of the normal working week, the relaxation of the weekend can allow the migraine to develop. Others get cluster migraines: months with no trouble at all and then continuous periods of migraine for days on end. Others get them in a seemingly random pattern, and some women get them closely related to their menstrual cycle. Often patients know some time beforehand that they are going to get an attack. They develop an aura of well-being or elation, or sometimes slight visual disturbances can herald the onset of an attack, whilst other people wake with them from their sleep.

The pain usually starts above or behind one eye or at the base of the skull, spreading over to one side of the head. The accompanying violent nausea and vomiting and the extreme sensitivity to light are symptoms of the classical migraine attack.

Naturopaths have constantly urged the holistic approach to this distressing illness and at least the orthodox medical profession is beginning to heed our advice as to the dietary and lifestyle changes necessary to cope with migraine.

Food

The chemical tyramine is thought to be one of the factors involved in adverse food reactions triggering migraine attacks. The common foods to be avoided are cheese, chocolate, red wine, sherry, port, citrus fruits, coffee and tea, although individual sufferers may have their own highly idiosyncratic adverse food reactions.

It's important for the migraine sufferer to keep a very careful diary for a period of time covering a number of migraine attacks. This way they may be able to identify foods, occupations, or work or leisure situations which can be implicated. Exercises to improve the flexibility of the neck and shoulder muscles, relaxation techniques and changes in diet are the first things to try. At the first sign of an attack, drink copious amounts of plain cold water, since this helps to trigger off the body's natural mechanism for eliminating fluids and may help to relieve the uneven pressures which are also thought to be triggers. During an attack, rest, quiet and the avoidance of light are all important. The application of a cold compress to the forehead and a hot compress to the nape of the neck also brings considerable relief.

Self-help with acupressure (see diagram on page 99) will help during an attack, but treatment from an acupuncturist will help to resolve some of the imbalances that occur, particularly in the treatment of the gall-bladder and liver meridians.

Herbal treatment with an infusion of lavender flowers and massaging lavender oil into the temples will help, and the use of the herb feverfew has been extremely successful in some cases. This can be obtained as tablets or you can eat the leaves, though take care to put them in a sandwich, since chewing feverfew leaves on their own can produce mouth ulcers. The homoeopathic remedy silica or lycopodium is useful and the use of relaxation techniques is essential.

Massage to relieve the extremes of muscular stress which are nearly always present is invaluable, particularly massage to the muscles of the neck, upper back, shoulders and face. Disturbances of the bite mechanism can produce unequal stresses on the joints at the angle of the jaw (the temporo-mandibular joints). Many dentists are now working with bite correction techniques and the chronic migraine sufferer should consult his or her dentist in order to make sure that there is not a bite abnormality.

A regular intake of a vitamin B complex together with calcium pantothenate (100 mg daily) is also helpful for many sufferers.

Osteopathic treatment is often a key factor in the long-term relief of migraine. Manipulative treatment to relieve the pressures on the nerve roots of the neck and to ensure good circulation through the arteries of the neck is a fundamental part of any overall approach to the treatment of migraine.

Whilst this is a distressing illness, there is hope. Many sufferers have obtained relief by a combination of the alternative therapies outlined above, but it must be remembered that migraine is not just a medical problem – it is also a severe social handicap, since it disrupts family and social life and can interfere with the patient's occupation. The inability to plan even the simplest outing due to fear of a migraine interrupting and disrupting these arrangements sometimes leads patients to become isolated and withdrawn. Support from family and friends and encouragement to attempt to participate in as full a life as possible are vital.

Insomnia

Everyone has occasional sleepless nights, although sleepless rarely means totally sleepless. Most of those who claim to have 'not slept a wink' have usually managed three or four hours of sleep if not more, but their conscious memories of the hours they spent tossing and turning are very powerful.

Many things can disturb the habitual pattern of a person's sleep. Pain is the major physical cause of sleeplessness, although most chronic insomniacs develop poor sleep patterns as a result of periods of stress, anxiety, depression or other emotional disturbances. Once disturbed it is sometimes extremely difficult to re-establish normal sleep patterns and the chronic insomniac's life takes on a depressing bleakness.

Many people worry needlessly about the amount of sleep they are getting, since as you get older your sleep requirements are certainly less and in any case the oft quoted eight hours is a myth. Many people live perfectly normal satisfactory lives on only four or five hours' sleep a night, and in fact there is evidence to show that 'short' sleepers tend to be the doers of our world.

The last resort in the treatment of sleep disorders should be medication. Rather you should first look to the causes – is your bed comfortable, is your bedroom too warm, are your nightclothes restricting your movement, is there enough fresh air, are there background noises which intrude into your subconscious? All these physical situations are easy to remedy.

The emotional disturbances are more difficult, but allowing someone to limp through life on crutches of sleeping pills, which especially in older people tend to aggravate any mental confusion which exists already, is a poor answer to one of life's common problems.

My advice to patients with sleep problems is not to lie in bed tossing, turning and worrying about not sleeping but to get up and do something – writing letters, doing the ironing, reading a book – anything which occupies the mind and helps to block out more disturbing thoughts and encourage natural fatigue is a good idea. Learning simple relaxation techniques, warm baths at bedtime (not hot) with relaxing herbal oils such as meadowsweet or orange blossom, will frequently help. Avoiding stimulants such as coffee, tea or caffeine-containing soft drinks and avoiding stimulating activities close to bedtime are all important. Watching the late night horror movie or reading a thrilling book is not the best remedy for someone who has problems sleeping.

A little gentle exercise after your evening meal is also a good idea. A walk, a cycle ride or just a few simple physical jerks will all help to encourage healthy fatigue.

As an alternative to the powerful sleeping pills, herbal remedies such as chamomile or lime blossom tea, Bio-Strath valerian formula or hop extracts all have a calmative effect. The homoeopathic remedies aconite, arnica or nux vomica are also recommended. Avoid having large meals late in the evening, encourage your partner to learn gentle massage techniques; and the use of 25 mg of vitamin B6 and dolomite tablets at bedtime is advisable.

Finally, hypnosis or the use of sleep-inducing music can also be tried since these seem to help many people.

Chronic insomnia is a miserable condition and strenuous efforts must be made to try to eradicate the cause as long-term lack of sleep does affect performance at work and social relationships.

Travel sickness

Travel sickness may be caused by any form of motion, in cars, aeroplanes, boats, swings, roundabouts, roller-coasters. The balance mechanism in the ear is responsible for transmitting signals to the brain which give information as to the movement of the head. When this information is different from that which the eyes can see, the brain becomes confused. In some people travel sickness follows. Nausea, vomiting, dizziness or faintness may all be symptoms.

Children are far more often affected than adults and most will grow out of the problem, although not all. There are many people who suffer travel sickness as passengers even though they can drive themselves with no problems.

Keeping children occupied on journeys, avoiding getting them too anxious or excited before setting out and obviously avoiding travelling either on top of a large meal or on a totally empty stomach are all important. If your children do get sick while travelling, make sure you carry plenty of drinks (not sweetened fizzy ones) as this will help to prevent the dehydration which may follow from long periods of vomiting.

Weak chamomile tea and chewing small pieces of crystallised ginger will help to alleviate the worst of the symptoms. The homoeopathic remedies cocculus and petroleum are both useful, and taking 25 mg of vitamin B6 (10 mg for children) half an hour before you travel and repeating the dose three hourly whilst travelling is also useful for many people. Ginger tea is the best of all natural remedies for motion sickness.

A little psychology is important when dealing with children who suffer from regular travel sickness. They very quickly associate the car or the bus with being sick, which creates enormous anxiety and apprehension and will almost certainly lead to repeated episodes. Reassuring the child, keeping its mind occupied and avoiding continual discussion of the child's travel sickness problem just before setting off on a journey will all help. Putting a bucket on the floor of the car the minute you open the door is not likely to encourage the child to travel well.

Neuralgia

This is the medical name for the severe pain which comes from some damage to a nerve. The most common forms are trigeminal neuralgia which affects the nerve of the face, sciatica which affects the sciatic nerve that travels from the lower part of the spine down the leg to the foot, and the severe pain of shingles which is caused by a virus living in the nerve tissue. Naturally it is important to treat the underlying cause of the problem which affects the nerve, but particularly in the case of the pain of shingles and trigeminal neuralgia it is very important to relieve the patient's discomfort.

The pain of shingles can be excruciating and can also last for a considerable length of time after the attack of shingles has passed. Without doubt the most effective treatment for this type of pain is the use of acupuncture administered by a qualified acupuncturist. Self-treatment using electrical machines which stimulate the acupuncture points can be helpful, although it is sometimes extremely difficult for patients to isolate the specific points which will help in their particular situation. Trigeminal neuralgia also responds well to acupuncture, but the question of the bite mechanism of the jaw must also be looked at since occasionally disturbances in the proper balance of the jaw when biting can cause uneven pressure which can lead to nerve irritation.

The use of alternating hot and cold compresses to the affected areas can also bring temporary relief and you should apply the hot pack for two minutes and the cold for 30 seconds. Continue for about 15 minutes.

Large doses of vitamin B1 starting at 500 mg daily and reducing the dose as the pain improves should also be tried.

The severe pain of herpes and trigeminal neuralgia can be extremely depressing to the patient and some patients may even become depressed to the point of suicide as a result of this intractable pain. In these very extreme situations the use of nerve-blocking agents or even of surgery to interrupt the pathway of the nervous impulses may be necessary, but in any case these people will need constant support and help and sympathetic understanding, since it is all too easy to dismiss them as simply moaning about their problem. No one who has not experienced these types of agonising pains can understand the torment which the unfortunate sufferers are having to put up with.

The seven ages of woman

Glowing health is every woman's birthright. The health that gives you bags of energy, and a positive outlook on life. The health that makes you look good because you feel good. The health that means a clear skin, bright eyes, glossy hair. The health that keeps you free from all the problems women are conditioned to expect – from acne to brittle bones, from morning sickness to postnatal depression, from PMS to menopausal problems.

The Well Woman's Eating Plan

The Well Woman's Eating Plan will show you how you can secure your birthright of good health. How you can fortify yourself against physical strain and nervous stress. How you can beef up your natural resistance to infection and disease. How you can kiss goodbye to the traditional woes of womanhood. How you can protect yourself against today's crop of disabling or life-threatening diseases – arthritis, osteoporosis, cancer, heart disease. And how you can keep your good looks for life without resorting to the beauty parlour or the plastic surgeon. This plan doesn't call for expensive pills or potions. It doesn't involve complicated diet sheets, expensive meal substitutes, or the latest food-fad regime.

The Well Woman's Eating Plan is the first positive guide to vitality eating, based on the nutritional Essential Foods you will learn to include in your weekly shopping basket. Everyday foods that you can buy in any supermarket, corner shop or street-market stall. Wonderful foods that can cost literally pennies – and yet in terms of your health are worth their weight in gold.

Vitality eating

Vitality means having both physical and mental vigour. They can both be yours if you follow the simple rules of vitality eating:

(1) Have a mixed diet of as many different foods as possible.
(2) Eat regular meals, and make sure that you have the time to enjoy and digest them.
(3) Eat plenty of fresh fruit, salads and vegetables, particularly the green leafy and yellow ones.

(4) Cultivate a taste for wholegrain cereals.
(5) Get most of your protein from fish, poultry, pulses, and less from meat, which should be as lean as possible.
(6) Have regular, but modest amounts of eggs, low-fat cheeses and other dairy products.
(7) Use plenty of fresh seeds, sprouted seeds and fresh, unsalted nuts, together with dried fruits. Add them to your meals and eat them as nourishing snacks.
(8) Drink plenty of fruit and vegetable juices, lots of water and only sensible quantities of tea, coffee and alcohol.
(9) Bread, pasta, rice and potatoes are very healthy. Have plenty of them, but watch what you do to them. Lashings of butter, cream sauces and the chip-pan are not part of this plan.
(10) Try to eat one-third of your daily food fresh and raw. For the other two-thirds, get into the kitchen. There is nothing as vital as home-cooked food, made from wholesome and nourishing ingredients. It is also a lot less expensive than take-aways, cans and TV dinners.

During each of the seven ages of woman, there are specific nutritional needs which are satisfied by the relevant Essential Foods. In each case the seven foods listed should be eaten every week. However, all the Essential Foods are important for all women. Whatever your age, get to know the entire list and use it as the foundation of your weekly shopping basket.

There is no need to feel guilty about the odd treat. As long as you are sticking to the spirit of this eating plan, you shouldn't become a food freak. There is nothing more boring than someone who takes their own food to a party, wrapped up in a brown paper bag. When your friends all go out, join in, enjoy whatever you eat and have a good time. A little of what you fancy does you good, so there's nothing wrong with an occasional chocolate éclair, doughnut, burger or chips, just so long as they are not your staple diet.

The teens

Your grown-up life starts here. Childhood is almost behind you, school no longer seems to stretch ahead forever, and already you may be enjoying a first taste of the independence that will soon be yours. You may be starting your first job – going on to more years of serious study – or training for a career.

These are years of growth, development and hormonal change, demanding the best possible nutrition. They are years, too, when you'll need all the energy you can get, to help you enjoy the fun – and cope with the stresses – of your busy, exciting, active life.

For growth, development and energy you need to follow the Vitality Eating rules on page 197. It's specially important for you to eat a proper breakfast; if you race for the bus every morning after no more than a snatched cup of coffee and half a piece of toast, the temptation to boost nose-diving blood-sugar levels with a mid-morning coffee or a Mars bar will be almost irresistible. Porridge is a great breakfast – you can make it in two or three minutes. It will give you vital minerals like iron, zinc, calcium – plus nerve-strengthening B-complex vitamins. Eat it with milk and a little honey for sweetening.

If lunch is sandwiches, make sure it's wholemeal bread; add a hard-boiled egg, cheese, tuna, tinned sardines or chicken for protein. And add plenty of chopped parsley too: just the stuff to give you a glowing, unblemished skin; cress is a good alternative. Round off your packed lunch with a carton of yoghurt – steer clear of those high in sugar and additives – and a piece of fruit: a banana, an apple or a pear.

Midday meals are likely to be a rush. So try to sit down to a sensible meal in the evening; eat it at leisure, and make sure it includes a green vegetable; spinach is super for you, so are celery, carrots, spring greens. Salad or at least one raw vegetable – is a must on the menu; it could be a couple of carrots scraped clean and cut into chunks, a crisp stick of celery, slivers of red or yellow peppers. Or try that USA favourite: a spinach salad with mushrooms thinly sliced into it, and a creamy garlicky dressing. If you don't want to be a social outcast, you'll find yourself heading for the Big Mac, the cokes and the chips with the rest of the gang. Enjoy yourself: but if there's a salad table – now in more and more fast food joints – help yourself; sample the vegeburgers at Wimpy's, and remember: one king-sized coke contains *fourteen* teaspoons of sugar!

The troublesome teens

Stress   Something teenagers know all about. Exams and the hours of anxious swotting that go with them, friendship problems, clashes with the family, first love with its agonies and ecstasies: all these can pile on the load. To cope with stress you need food that's rich in B-complex vitamins; wholegrain cereals – including the oats in your porridge – liver, meat, chicken, fish, leafy green vegetables.

Wholegrain cereals   – Brown rice, wholemeal bread – will supply the zinc you need for growth and a gorgeous skin; iron for energy and mental staying-power; calcium and magnesium for beautiful bones.

Low energy   Shouldn't be a problem for teenagers, but it often is, and girls are specially at risk, because of the monthly drain on their vital iron reserves. Make sure you're getting plenty of iron in your diet – not just from the classic liver, but also from egg yolks, spinach, lentils, nuts and seeds. Did you know, by the way, that drinking tea or coffee at the same time will hinder your body's ability to absorb that iron? Vitamin C has the opposite effect, luckily; eat a piece of fruit or drink an orange juice at the same meal.

Excess weight Often worries teenagers. But whatever you do, don't cut down on the sensible food you need for growth and energy; and steer clear of those dangerous lettuce-leaf-and-black-coffee diets; they can seriously damage your health. Instead, just remember that the key factors are likely to be excess *fat* and excess *sugar* in your diet. There's an awful lot of fat – and the dodgy saturated kind too – in most processed foods: sausages, burgers, salami, meat pies, chips, crisps, ice-cream. Sweet fizzy drinks really pile on the sugar; a 3½ oz milk chocolate bar contains a staggering 56.5 g – that's about a dozen lumps of sugar! – and over 500 calories. Watch breakfast cereals too. If your sweet tooth aches for comfort, have a banana, an apple, some dried fruit, or lovely fresh dates instead; they'll give you an instant energy lift-off.

Anorexia Can sneak up on you if you become too obsessive about weight and start cutting out mineral-rich foods. The vital mineral here is zinc, lack of which can zap taste-buds and destroy appetite; good sources are shrimps, liver, lean meat, the wheatgerm that's missing from white bread, sesame and pumpkin seeds; mackerel, cheese and green vegetables.

Acne and other skin problems Will take care of themselves if you watch fat and sugar intake. Your best friend, though, is the colour *green* which should always be on the menu, even if it's only a sprig of parsley. Green in vegetables and herbs means lots of beta-carotene, which your body will process into Vitamin A – vital for healthy skin and clear eyes. And green also means lots of chlorophyll, which has a marvellously cleansing, nourishing and anti-infection action on your skin.

To keep you streamlined, clear-skinned and full of energy, finally, you need exercise – and that doesn't mean swaying gently in a smoke-filled disco. Pick the exercise you really enjoy – basketball, running, swimming, tennis, a brisk country walk – and build it into your life.

Essential foods
Dates To satisfy your sweet tooth. They'll supply badly needed iron, too, and they're high in potassium.

Eggs   The original low-calorie convenience food. Eggs are a good source of protein, supplying around 6 g a time.

Lentils   These are rich in protein – over 23 g in 100 g – and if you eat vitamin-C rich food at the same meal, you'll also absorb their valuable iron and zinc.

Oranges   Eat a whole fresh orange at the start of a meal, and you'll up your intake of iron, calcium and other useful minerals on the day's menu.

Porridge   You couldn't have a better start to the day than this traditional Scottish breakfast.

Pumpkin seeds   Eat them for valuable B vitamins, for iron, for zinc and for unsaturated fatty acids.

Spinach   This owes its deep, dark green colour to its high content of chlorophyll and it also has a high beta-carotene content.

Parsley   Rich in vitamins A and C, as well as iron.

The twenties

You're on your own now; and your life is what *you* make it. You're already settled into a job; you've left home for a place of your own; you have your own friends and social life.

This is the age of romance, when the man in your life can swallow up most of your time and attention. It can also be the age of broken hearts . . . unless you're married already, and trying to get to grips with domestic chores as well as a job.

But married or still single, you'll find the days are never long enough for all you want to cram into them. And your diet should be supplying handsome insurance against stress of every kind – trials at work, romance gone awry, too many late nights, and too many skimpy meals eaten in a rush. Turn to the Vitality Eating Rules on page 197: cut them out, pin them up in the first ever kitchen you can call your own – and stick to them.

Office lunches can be a healthy treat these days: most supermarkets sell a range of made-up salads, starring carrots, coleslaw, apples, celery, nuts, brown rice. Add a glass of milk or a carton of yoghurt, a piece of fruit – and you'll be ready for the most taxing afternoon.

Bedsitter cooking can degenerate into endless snacks of bread, cheese and canned soup. Make sure you don't run out of the basics: potatoes, carrots, onions, a good olive oil, lemons, sliced wholewheat bread, garlic. Stock up on salad-stuff – celery, red and yellow peppers, watercress, a box of cress, spring onions – that will last two or three days in the fridge. Keep supplies of eggs, low-fat yoghurt, cottage cheese, skimmed milk, nuts, seeds in the fridge too; a bowl of fruit on the table – apples, bananas, oranges; and in the store cupboard, cans of tuna, sardines (canned in olive oil please) tomatoes, sugar-free baked beans, brown rice, pasta and dried herbs. Then you'll always be able to whip up a healthy square meal - soup, salad, pasta, risotto – no matter how tired you are.

Cooking should be a pleasure as well as a necessity – and it can be a wonderful way to unwind at the end of a stressful day. Master a few survival recipes, so that you can rustle up a decent meal in the evening. Everybody – male or female – should know how to make a good rich vegetable soup. Teach yourself, too, how to use nature's seasonings instead of loads of pepper, salt and bottled sauces; thyme gives a wonderful flavour to stews and fish, and when you cook a chicken, stuff it with a big bunch of thyme; this natural antibiotic will help protect you against infections, too. Experiment with some of the new natural seasonings; Schwartz have a range of peppers flavoured with mixtures of the healthgiving and tasty herbs, another alternative to salt.

Problems of the tough twenties

Menstrual problems Can be a real drag at this age; cramps, irritability, tension, nausea and bloating are among the monthly trials which so many women seem to regard as inevitable. Far from being inevitable, however, menstrual problems are as much an index of ill health as muddy skin or lank hair, and just as avoidable. It's Kitchen Therapy to the rescue once more. Eat plenty of wholegrain cereals, nuts and seeds – particularly almonds, oats, sesame and sunflower seeds: they'll supply the magnesium, the B-complex vitamins, the vital vitamin E and the iron that will help resolve your problems. Bananas are an Essential Food for you; rich in vitamin B6 and iron, their high potassium content helps your kidneys cope with water retention problems. They're the dieter's friend too – wonderfully filling and nourishing, but still only around 90 calories for an average-size fruit.

Stress For the twenties this often takes the form of too many late nights, hectic romantic involvements, financial worries, work problems and skimpy fast-food meals. Eat lots of B-complex-rich wholegrain cereals – wholewheat bread, brown rice, oats – to help you cope: they'll supply a rich diet for the nerves, and give you extra stamina too, in the shape of calcium, iron, magnesium. If the jar of instant coffee is always at hand at home or in the office, ration

yourself; too much tea or coffee can make you *very* nervous –
though you may not realise why. Try one of the many coffee-
substitutes found in health food shops; Swiss Bambu is our
favourite. Apart from zapping nerves, excess caffeine will stop your
body absorbing half the good minerals you may be feeding it; for
maximum uptake, eat fruit or fresh vitamin-C rich vegetables and
salads at the same meal.

Smoking and drinking   If you acquired these habits in your teens,
to prove how grown-up you were, get a grip on them now. Any
veteran smoker can tell you – it gets harder all the time to give up!
The same goes for excess drinking; it's now known that the female
liver has fairly low resistance to alcohol, so don't think you can
drink with the boys and get away with it. Both smoking and alcohol
generate free radical activity – now known to give you wrinkles!
Instead of a packet of cigarettes, keep a packet of sunflower seeds in
your desk drawer to nibble at; they're little powerhouses of good
nutrition. Don't be browbeaten into drinking for social reasons;
these days, mineral water is seen on the chic-est restaurant tables.
Instead of alcohol, drink a non-alcoholic 'cooler' of apple or
pineapple juice with bubbly mineral water, or the terrific new
vegetable juice cocktails they sell in supermarkets, chilled and
spiked with lemon. And if you order a glass of white wine – have a
mineral water next round and drink spritzers the rest of the evening.

Skin problems   Like acne, these can be even more agonising in your
twenties than in your teens; your appearance is vitally important to
you. Don't panic: try to keep one day a week when you eat nothing
but fruit or vegetables, to give your whole system a good clean-out.
And high on the list should be avocadoes; research in Israel has
shown that they help reconstitute the springy collagen that keeps skin
young. Other vital skin-foods are all the crucifer vegetables
– including cauliflower, broccoli and cabbage; chlorophyll-rich
spinach and watercress; and all brightly coloured fruit, especially
peaches, nectarines and apricots. They're loaded with beta-
carotene, which is great for your skin.

Overweight   Will likewise respond to a fruit and vegetable 'fast'. If
it's a real problem, keep a food diary – write down every single thing
you eat or drink – for a week; work out how to 'lose' 500 calories
daily of either fat or sugar; and force yourself to exercise briskly –
enough to get up a bit of a sweat – at least four times a week. Splurge
on a ravishing new leotard, and commit yourself to a regular
exercise or dance class with a friend; be an energetic disco dancer;
or walk part of the way to and from work. Brisk exercise 'tunes'
your metabolism so you burn up fat faster.

Essential foods

Avocados   They're extremely nutritious – highly digestible – and wonderfully filling for their calorie count – around 160 for half a pear.

Bananas   These are high in potassium, for healthy hearts, and they're full of a useful fibre called pectin.

Carrots   A single carrot will supply your vitamin A needs for an entire day.

Cauliflower   Cauliflower supplies silicon – for strong bones, healthy hair, firm skin.

Potatoes   These are good news for the intelligent slimmer: even a whopper of a baked potato, crispy skin and all, is only around 200 calories.

Sunflower seeds   Packed with wonderful nutrients – vitamins, minerals, unsaturated fats, protein.

Tuna   This contains omega-3 fats, the good fats which have a strongly protective action on the heart.

Thyme   This has powerful anti-viral and anti-bacterial properties.

Pregnancy

The folk-lore of pregnancy is a minefield of myth and magic, and a catalogue of 'dos and don'ts'. The first step on the road to a safe, happy and successful pregnancy is to ignore conflicting advice from well-meaning friends and relatives and all the old-wives' tales. Rely on your own common sense and make sure that you understand as much about this wonderful event as possible. Don't be afraid to ask your doctor or consultant about things which worry you.

Of course, there are problems and risks, and you may not feel 100 per cent for every single day of the nine months. But you can swing the odds in your favour. You can combat the morning sickness, reduce the tiredness, avoid the excessive weight gain and see that your growing baby is getting the best possible nourishment, while at the same time protecting your own future health. You can even do something about the seemingly inevitable indigestion, constipation, varicose veins and piles. It's a simple question of how, what and when, you eat; the right balance of rest and exercise; a positive outlook and bags of confidence.

Pregnant problems

A question of weight   The easiest thing for you to control during pregnancy is your weight. It is also one of the most important, both for you and the baby. Even in the perfect pregnancy there are some discomforts to put up with and if you pile on the pounds they will be worse. Back ache, heartburn, piles, varicose veins, stretch marks and tiredness; all will be worse if you are too heavy. Serious problems are more common in the really overweight. But your baby is the prime concern. A 20–30 lb gain is what to aim for over the nine months. Avoid crash diets; the first three months is the time for good calories and the vital nutrients which the growing baby needs. If you find your weight has got to the limit after six months, then the last three months is no time for panic measures. Brain development needs protein and calories.

It is easy to do it right, gain 30 lb and have a baby at around the ideal of 6½–8½ lb. On the other hand a junk food diet that adds 3½ stone to you may result in an underweight 5 lb baby, which will be more at risk.

Eat at least four of the Essential Foods each day, a varied mixture of the healthy, low-fat, high nutrient Essential Foods in other sections, and aim for no more than 2400 calories and 60 g of protein a day. A grilled herring supplies 24 g, three walnuts 2 g, four table-spoons of brown rice 4.4 g, three thin slices of liver around 25 g, one egg 8 g, one carton of low-fat yoghurt 7.5 g.

Morning sickness   Most women can master this misery. Eat a little nourishing snack before bedtime so that your stomach is not empty. Keep a secret store on your bedside table for midnight feasts. Oatmeal biscuits, crispbreads, walnuts, raisins, sesame seeds and a bottle of plain mineral water. Make sure that you have a drink of peppermint tea, lime flower tea with a little fresh ginger grated into it or weak ordinary tea, with a little honey and no milk, and a plain unsweetened biscuit as soon as you wake. It is best if brought to your bed so that you have it before getting up.

Anaemia and Toxaemia   You must cut down the risks of these serious complications of pregnancy. Iron and protein are the key foods. Include at least two portions of the green leafy veg and three protein foods each day. Magnesium is a key mineral here, and the richest sources are chickpeas, kidney beans, cashew nuts and mackerel.

Constipation   This is so easy to prevent, and yet causes more discomfort than many of the other problems. Tackle it before it is there, by increasing the amount you drink. Have at least 3 pints of fluid each day, not too much of which is tea or coffee. Keep off the fizzy drinks and watch out for the high natural sugar content of even the pure fruit juices. They should be diluted 50/50 with water. Brown rice, wholemeal bread, dried fruits, vegetables, potatoes cooked with their skins, baked beans and porridge, are great sources of natural fibre which keep everything on the move. *Don't* sprinkle spoonsful of bran over your plate, it prevents you from absorbing calcium and iron. Do eat at least three high fibre foods daily.

Varicose veins and piles   These are not an inevitable fact. They are both linked with constipation, so avoiding it protects you from them. Vitamin E is essential, get it from kiwi fruit, herring, tuna, extra virgin olive oil, nuts and tinned tomatoes. Garlic and onions are also great protectors of your circulatory system. Have two of these foods daily. Avoid standing, take plenty of walks or other exercise, and if there is a family history of varicose veins, wear good support tights or stockings.

Exhaustion   You will need as much energy as you can muster for the new baby, so lots of energy during this nine months is vital. Complex carbohydrates are much better at providing it than sugars and refined starches. Brown rice, wholemeal bread, lentils, beans, nuts and good cereals like muesli, porridge, Weetabix or Shredded Wheat, are the first choice. Eggs, fish, poultry, lean meat and dairy products supply the protein that you need.

Acid indigestion   So-called 'heartburn' is prevented by eating a little and often. This is most important in the later stages as it stops the build-up of pressure on the diaphragm. It is this pressure which stretches the muscle that keeps the food pipe closed, and so allows the acid in the stomach to flow upward and cause the pain. Use plenty of cloves in your cooking, avoid the frying pan, chew food well and don't eat on the hoof.

High blood pressure   The most dreaded of all the pregnancy problems. Keep yours in check by following the advice on weight, varicose veins, anaemia and constipation. Eat lots of herrings, other oily fish and all the seven Essential Foods for this section. Regular exercise is essential, coping with stress using relaxation exercise, yoga, meditation, and organising your life so as to avoid overcommitment will all help. Garlic and onions are of special value.

Essential foods
Apples   These neutralise acidity produced by indigestion. They

contain pectin, a fibre that keeps the bowels functioning, and lowers cholesterol.

Broccoli   This is a rich source of vitamins A and C. It also provides iron which is easily absorbed by the body, and is a good supplier of calcium and potassium.

Brown rice   Provides many of the B vitamins, some fibre, iron, potassium and protein.

Herrings   These are a fine source of vitamins A, D and B. They also contain iodine, selenium, phosphorus, potassium, iron and calcium. Most importantly during pregnancy, they supply the omega-3 fatty acids.

Kiwi fruit   These give you twice as much vitamin C as an orange, more fibre than an apple, as much vitamin E as an avocado and lots of potassium, a lack of which can lead to fatigue and poor digestion.

Onions   These are good for the heart and circulation.

Walnuts   Are high in protein, B vitamins, calcium, potassium, phosphorus, zinc and iron.

Cloves   This aromatic spice is a great aid to digestion. It reduces nausea, flatulence and dyspepsia.

Motherhood

There's nothing else in life quite like it: the joy of that moment when you first hold your newborn baby in your arms. Suddenly all those long dreary months of waiting seem worthwhile.

But as any mother can tell you, motherhood can be tough going – and the first time round especially so. For a start, you'll be more tired than you ever imagined possible; you'll *never* get as much sleep as you need. Even the simplest household chores can suddenly seem overwhelming; a cross word will reduce you to tears; and you'll wonder despairingly how on earth other women ever cope with it all. Once the baby is a toddler, you'll get a decent night's sleep at last – but you'll need it to cope with an active, demanding 2-year-old. And the average mother of 4- and 5-year-olds will thank you with tears in her eyes, if you can arrange just a couple of hours of freedom for her.

When life is so hectic and demanding, preparing proper meals for yourself may seem a chore you can forget about. Instead, you'll go for the temporary 'lift' of a cup of tea and a couple of sweet biscuits; and later on, something out of a tin or the remains of the nursery lunch will do. What they can't and won't do, however, is give you the strength, the nervous resilience and the sheer stamina that Vitality Eating supplies. Study the rules on page 197. Don't shortchange yourself; your health is vital. Not just for you but for the whole family.

Your midday meal doesn't have to be a lot of fuss; a carton of low-fat yoghurt – stir in a little honey, some nuts; a baked potato or a wholemeal roll with a piece of cheese, a couple of sticks of celery and an apple. That's a beautifully balanced meal that will keep you going for hours. Between-meals snacks? Dried fruit – especially *apricots* – will give you a real energy lift. Eat liver once a week; otherwise, cut down on red meat and spend the money on extra fresh fruit and vegetables, especially cabbages, watercress and spring greens, which will raise your resistance to infection and stress.

Post-natal depression This may seem like a state of mind – but the right diet can help banish it for good. First, get more rest and sleep at all costs, even if it means a messy house, and no clean shirts for your husband. Your diet should star the whole-grains – oats, wholewheat, brown rice – for the stress-proofing that their B-complex vitamins will give you; yoghurt for calcium; and green leafy vegetables for magnesium, a nutrient badly needed by the stressed nervous system. Zinc is another vital nutrient, and it's specially likely to be deficient in mothers who took iron supplements in pregnancy, as the two minerals need to be in balance. Liver, shrimps, beef, cheese, sardines and wholemeal bread all supply zinc. For an extra shot in the arm, take a daily tablespoon of dried brewer's yeast; blend it with a carton of low-fat yoghurt, a banana, and half a glass of orange juice for a delicious drink that's also a complete meal in a glass. Brewer's yeast is loaded with B-vitamins and vital minerals, including zinc.

Stress Non-stop demands on your attention can be a particularly exhausting form of stress, which in turn lowers your resistance to infection of any kind. To beef up your immune defences, eat foods rich in vitamins A and C: brightly coloured fruits like oranges, *grapefruit* – especially the pink ones – peaches, nectarines, blackcurrants and all other berries. The famous Swiss, Dr Bircher-Benner – who cured illnesses with a diet high in raw foods – used to tell his patients: 'Eat green leaves every day.' It's advice you couldn't do better than follow. Cabbage, watercress, spring greens, spinach, all kinds of lettuce: they're richly protective, supplying chlorophyll – wonderful for your skin, and anti-bacterial – as well as vitamin A, and useful minerals like calcium and magnesium.

Overweight   You may feel that by rights you should be worn to a shadow – yet you may actually be overweight, and listless with it. Sweet snacks that are high in calories, fats and sugar, but poor in real nutrition and in fibre – the classic coffee and doughnut, or tea and bun – are among the commonest reasons. Have a healthy snack instead: a piece of fruit, a handful of raisins or a carton of yoghurt with a little honey stirred in. And remember that excess fat and refined carbohydrate put a heavy workload on your digestive system – while lack of fibre can bring it all to a grinding halt. Poor digestion itself can lead to much more serious health problems in the long run – cancer, arthritis and heart disease among them. In the short term it will stop you ever feeling on peak form.

Fatigue   This is what makes young mothers tense and irritable. Fatigue doesn't leave you feeling very sexy, and you won't have much energy to spend on looking attractive either. At times like these, remember the stores of energy and nutritional wealth packed into tiny seeds. In the traditional medicine of the Middle East, sesame seeds have always been associated with enhanced sexual energy and prowess. Eat them in ready-made purée form; called tahini, every health food shop – and many ethnic grocers – stock it. Or at any delicatessen you can buy hummus, the savoury dip made from tahini and chickpeas, to enjoy with flat wholewheat pitta bread, and chunks of raw vegetables. The zinc in sesame seeds will also do wonders for your skin.

The fragrant herb basil is a wonderful tonic for fatigue. Italians wouldn't make a tomato salad without it; and *pesto* sauce, from the delicatessen, made with lots of basil and pinenuts, is an extra-delicious ready-made sauce for pasta.

Both fatigue and weight problems will respond to active exercise, out in the open air. Pram-pushing may give you the fresh air and sunshine; but you need something just a little more strenuous two to three times a week. Swimming is the ideal exercise for you and babies love it too! Make it a family outing that you'll all enjoy.

Essential foods

Apricots   Are rich in beta-carotene that your body converts into vitamin A. Dried apricots are rich in iron, but wash them thoroughly in warm water to remove the sulphur dioxide used as a preservative.

Cabbage   Can help you cope with stress, anaemia, fatigue and infection.

Grapefruit This is loaded with vitamins A and C – the pink kind are even higher in A.

Liver This is crammed with vitamin A, B-complex, and so much iron and zinc. Zinc is especially important if you're suffering from post-natal depression.

Sesame seeds All seeds are regenerating, vital foods, specially useful to help you meet the demands of a rushed and busy life.

Watercress This contains a natural antibiotic. It's also rich in the vitamin A precursor beta-carotene and iron.

Yoghurt Not only is it twice as easy to digest as milk; it contains *acidophilus* bacteria which will re-create a healthy balance in your gut. It's great fast food – all you need is a spoon!

Basil This has a mild calming action. The old herbalists used it to help restore regular periods, and as a remedy for nervous headaches.

The vital thirties

These are the years of your beautiful prime. You'll never have more natural energy than you have now; your looks have the appeal of maturity as well as the glow of youth; you have grown-up confidence and poise.

But sometimes you really wish you were Superwoman. The man in your life probably expects you to be a faultless housekeeper, a crack cook, and the gorgeous girl he first fell for, all rolled into one. The job gets tougher as you climb the promotion ladder. If you have children you'll find they need more and more of your time, love and attention as they head for the troublesome teens.

Moreover, if you're running a home *and* job *and* raising a family, then you'll sometimes wonder how you got yourself into all this.

But don't reach for the quick fix of coffee, stiff drink or cigarette; and don't fall on the sweet snacks for a quick energy lift that will let you down later – as well as aggravating any weight problems you may have. There are much better ways to keep you firing on all cylinders.

Above all, don't be tempted to save time and trouble by skipping meals, or lunching off a couple of coffees and a Kit-Kat, or serving up endless microwaved TV dinners because it's much too much trouble to cook, and you feel tired to death.

For these rich, demanding years of your life, only first-class nourishment is good enough; you can't be Superwoman on anything but Superfood.

Turn to the Vitality Eating rules on page 197, to remind yourself what good nutrition is all about. Wholegrains, fresh fruits and vegetables, raw salads, fresh herbs sprouting on the windowsill are basics. So are yoghurt, milk, cheese and supplies of fresh nuts – preferably still in their shells – and seeds stored in the fridge.

If daily shopping is out of the question, go for the vegetables that will stay fresh happily for a few days: potatoes, carrots, onions, stored out of the light, in a cool place, in brown paper bags; and in the fridge supplies of salad-stuffs like sweet peppers, celery, fennel and watercress. In a dark corner of your kitchen, devote space to sprouting seeds: a helping of pure vitality that's organically grown, morning-fresh, additive-free – and cheap with it.

Build your vitality

Beat PMS   You must do something to overcome this draining and depressing problem. It is not uncommon for it to get worse after you have children, and it will add further to the stresses of this extra hectic period of your life. Fight the craving for sugar and chocolate bars. Sweet fruits like grapes and melon will help. So, too, will dried fruit and almonds. Increase your intake of vitamin B6 from eggs, oily fish like salmon and sardines, wholegrain cereals and bananas. You will need more zinc and magnesium from pumpkin seeds, liver, shellfish, chickpeas, kidney beans and mackerel. Cut down on tea, coffee, alcohol and sugar.

Look after your heart   Now is the time to take a real interest in the affairs of your heart. This is a time of growing responsibility, career, husband, children or all three. You are likely to be under more stress and pressure, to have less time to look after yourself and your diet. This is not the time to let things slide. Ensure your future heart health by eating plenty of high fibre foods, lots of oily fish such as sardines, vegetable proteins like millet, buckwheat and beans. Foods rich in vitamins A and C such as cantaloupe melon, dark green leafy vegetables and as many onions and as much garlic as you can. Use extra virgin olive oil on salads. Cut down animal fats, salt, refined carbohydrates and drink modest amounts of alcohol – around fourteen glasses of wine or pub measures of spirits or half pints of beer, as an absolute maximum, per week. Do take some form of regular exercise, which should be weight bearing.

Let your skin bloom   All-round good nutrition is the foundation of a good skin. No amount of expensive lotions and potions will compensate for a bad diet. You need lots of vitamin A, from

211

carrots, melon, spinach, nectarines, apricots, kiwi fruit and liver. Chlorophyll from all green leafy vegetables, vitamin E from seeds, nuts, cold pressed seed oils and avocados. Eat millet for extra silicon. And don't forget dandelion leaves and celery with its green tops, both of which improve elimination of waste products.

Stress and super resistance   You do not have the time to get ill right now, so what can you do to boost your own resistance to infection and disease? Even if you are making the effort to eat well, much of the food you buy is likely to be missing out on some of the vital ingredients. That is why you need to have a regular daily input of the Essential Foods that are extra rich in vitamin C, zinc, vitamin A, and the B complex. Grapes, citrus fruits, apricots, black-currants, pineapple, broccoli, peppers, onions, oats, wheatgerms, almonds, sprouted seeds, yoghurt, chicken livers (free range), eggs, poultry, game and sardines, mackerel and herrings. These should form your staple diet. Stress is a great destroyer of defence mechanisms; it needs all the same nutritional help, plus lots of celery which is one of nature's great calmers. Drink lime flower tea with some honey in it to help you relax, and try any form of relaxation exercise. Yoga, meditation or self-hypnosis work well.

Bones matter now   The menopause may seem a long way off, but what happens now will determine the state of your bones in thirty years' time. You must start building up your calcium deposits. To do that you need calcium, vitamin D and sunlight. Each day you should eat a selection of at least three of the following foods: sardines (eat the bones), spinach, low-fat cheese, yoghurt, seeds, nuts, celery, turnips, cabbage, chickpeas, herring, tuna, eggs, dried fruits, brown rice, buckwheat and half a pint of skimmed milk. You must get as much daylight as you can. That does not mean cooking on the beach for two weeks of the year, but getting out into the fresh air and light for some time each day. It is vital that you start exercising now as well. Weight bearing makes the bones stronger. Walking, active sport like tennis, squash, badminton, netball, running or jogging are good for the bones. Cycling and swimming will get your heart working, but won't add to the strength of your skeleton.

Essential foods

Almonds   These are a very concentrated food, rich in protein, good fats, zinc, magnesium, potassium and iron, as well as some B vitamins.

Celery   This is a good nerve tonic as it contains a lot of calcium. Its diuretic properties have been known for centuries and you can eat it to get rid of fluid retention around period time.

Cheese   This is a rich source of protein, calcium and phosphorus, as well as the B vitamins. Lots of vitamin A, together with some vitamin D and E. Feta, Edam, cottage cheese and curd cheese are low in fats.

Grapes   These are easy to digest, and uniquely nourishing and fortifying.

Melon   The cantaloupe and ogen are rich sources of vitamin A.

Sardines   These are every woman's friend – rich in protein, vitamins D and B12, calcium and well-absorbed iron and zinc.

Sprouted seeds   The most live, pure and nutritious food you can grow on your windowsill.

Sage   A powerful healing and antiseptic herb.

Menopause

There is no need to dread the onset of the menopause. It is not a disease, nor some abnormality. It is nature's way of preventing pregnancy when it is no longer a good idea.

There are symptoms of the menopause which can be unpleasant and distressing, those which may lead to medical problems, and those which can be the cause of severe depression. You can improve and control them all. It helps to start your action plan before you reach the critical years (see The Vital Thirties), but if you are there now, don't despair. It is still possible to make dramatic changes in the way you feel, all that's needed is a close look at your eating habits.

Hot flushes, weight gain, headaches, brittle bones, skin problems, depression, sexual difficulties and an increased risk of heart disease are the most common results of the menopause – they can all be improved by the Essential Foods.

Beat the menopause miseries

Hot flushes   The lower levels of the hormone oestrogen are the main cause. Stress, being very thin, wearing tight-fitting clothes, as well as room temperature can all make things worse. Vitamin E can help a lot. The best sources are sesame seeds and their oil, sunflower seed oil, almonds, wholemeal bread, dark green leafy vegetables, eggs and cheese. Make sure that at least three of these are on your daily menu.

Weight gain   This is a regular anxiety of the menopause. Use all the Essential Foods of the Well Woman's Eating Plans, with a lot of those in this section, to construct the weekly menu. Avoid visible fats as much as you can. Make sure that you get some exercise each day. Oats, cooked any way you like, are an aid to weight loss, as they help elimination. They are also a satisfying and filling food.

Headaches   Often related to the hot flushes, and also to the stress and tension that arise at this time. Beetroot is excellent here, but don't forget the leaves and red stems. Use both root and leaf, raw in salads, dressed with sunflower seed oil, lemon juice and sprinkled with sesame seeds. Beetroot improves the oxygen-carrying ability of the blood and is rich in iron.

Brittle bones   Do not believe the experts who tell you that it is too late to do anything about your bones, once you have reached the menopause. You can still help yourself to better bones: more calcium, magnesium, zinc and vitamin D; more sunlight and more weight-bearing exercise. These will all help. So look to your shopping basket. It must contain plenty of spring greens, green, red and yellow peppers, nectarines, or any of the dark green or yellow fruits or vegetables, chickpeas, pumpkin seeds, sardines, yoghurt and low-fat cheese. Eat at least three of these each day.

Skin problems   These are also caused by a drop in the oestrogen levels. Vitamins A and E will both help. Eat plenty of the dark green and yellow vegetables and fruits. Apricots and pumpkins are good. Avocado has a special place here, and you ought to eat two a week. Yoghurt, used as a skin cream, is a good idea, too.

Depression   After the hot flushes, this is the commonest of problems. Calcium, magnesium and the amino acid tryptophan, will all do you good. Get them from dairy products, spinach, chickpeas and sesame seeds. The B vitamins are vital, and you'll find these in liver, oily fish, wholegrain cereals, eggs, spinach and yeast extracts. You must have at least two of these each day. Exercise stimulates the production of adrenalin, which makes you feel a lot better, so try to make time for physical exertion every day.

Sexual difficulties   The drop in oestrogen affects the secretions of the vagina, and the quality of the tissue in the sexual organs. An active, regular sex life will delay these changes considerably. It is likely that many women will spend their later years alone, since most will survive their husbands. For them, and the single women, it does not matter whether the sexual stimulation is the result of intercourse or masturbation, it's having regular orgasms that counts. The vitamin A and E foods are essential, so make sure of at least two servings daily from oily fish, liver, apricots, spinach, carrots or other green and yellow veg. Vegetable oils, nuts, seeds, eggs and wholegrain cereals are all good. Ginseng is a must here, and for all of the menopausal symptoms. It enhances the action of oestrogens, so making the most of what your body is producing. It also has an oestrogen-like activity of its own. Take some on a regular daily basis.

Heart disease   Young women have a much lower risk of heart disease than men, for whom it is the commonest cause of premature death. Once the menopause is reached, women are just as likely to suffer this scourge of the Western world. Good nutrition now becomes even more vital. Follow the rules for vitality eating, on page 197, and you will be on the right track. Vitamin C is important as it reduces the risk of blood clots; eat plenty of red, green and yellow peppers, kiwi fruit, oranges and blackcurrants. Onions and garlic are good for reducing cholesterol, as is lecithin from eggs, soya beans and liver.

Essential foods

Sesame seeds   Very rich in protein, iron and zinc.

Red, green and yellow peppers   These are an excellent source of vitamin C, but the red and yellow ones also provide a good supply of vitamin A.

Beetroot   A traditional medicine for building up the run-down and convalescent. The iron content is good, and its absorption enhanced by the vitamin C, so it is a valuable addition to the menopause diet.

Oats   A good source of easily digested protein, B-complex vitamins, some vitamin E, calcium, magnesium, potassium and silica.

Spring greens   These are a real life saver during the menopause, containing potassium, calcium and iron, and a very rich source of vitamins A and C.

Chickpeas   A super menopause food as they supply protein, vitamins A, C and some of the B complex. Also calcium, iron, zinc, potassium, magnesium and phosphorus.

Nectarines   These supply the essential vitamin A.

Ginseng   This has a powerful tonic and stimulating effect, so is great if you feel a bit down. Take it as a tea in small but regular doses.

The golden years

Today you can expect to live at least till the age of 75. It seems strange that at the turn of this century the lifespan of women was no more than 50. The menopause hardly existed, and the prospect of another 25 golden years was not even a pipe dream. Now, with the help of the Essential Foods, you can enjoy this bonus to the full.

There is no need to suffer in silence, with the stiff, aching joints of rheumatism and arthritis. Indigestion and insomnia are not inevitable. Lost concentration and memory can be pushed aside. The spectre of heart and circulatory disease need not haunt you. After all, if you have got this far, you can't have got it totally wrong.

The brain loses cells as it grows older, the muscles lose some strength, the joints some flexibility, the digestion some tolerance and the eyes and ears some sharpness. These are the normal process of living. You are not just what you eat, you *are* what you absorb from what you eat. You are also what you think and feel. You must have a positive attitude to life, and not let your age stop you from doing anything that you wish. This is the time for maximum nutrition, and it is geared to foods that supply the most nutrients in the most digestible form. You need high intakes of vitamins and minerals, B complex, A, C and E – the super nutrients that protect and nourish each cell in the body.

Survival for the senior citizen

Memory and concentration The B vitamins are essential for the proper working of the entire nervous system, and that includes the brain. A steady level of blood sugar is another factor; to achieve this you must eat regular meals, which supply enough starches and natural sugars. Liver, chicken and sardines are most important. Dried fruits, like dates, figs and apricots, should be eaten every day, as they contain the minerals which prevent the body from taking up aluminium – now thought to be a factor in causing senility. Vitamin C is also needed for this effect, so eat strawberries and citrus fruit.

Joint problems To keep rheumatism and athritis at bay, eat plenty of turnips, and their leafy tops. They increase the elimination of uric acid from the system, which aggravates joint problems. Strawberries have a cleansing effect and are also good for the joints. To keep up your muscle strength you need protein. Chicken is a good source, and you can make a soup from the leftovers. Put in lots of green veg, and roots, so that you have a highly nutritious broth

216

which will keep you warm as well as fed. All the oily fish are important; have them three times a week.

Digestion   You must eat at regular times, and sensible quantities. Four smaller meals a day are better. Even if you are alone, lay the table, put a sprig of flowers on it, and make mealtimes special. Eat slowly and chew well (look after your teeth, and see a dentist at least once a year if you have your own, every other year if you have dentures, as your mouth can change and make them a bad fit). Lentils are an excellent form of protein, easy to digest without causing wind. Avoid fatty foods, and eat some chicory each day to stimulate your liver. Pears are a good end to a meal. They have some fibre, vitamin C, and lots of potassium. This can be important if you are taking diuretic (water) pills.

Constipation   Less exercise, poor diet and too much tea and coffee can soon produce this problem. Don't let it happen to you. Wholegrain bread and cereals, dried fruits, millet, greens and plenty of fresh fruit and salads are needed. Drink plenty of water. If you worry about getting up in the night, then make sure you take a glassful as soon as you wake, another during the morning, and at least two more before teatime. Add lots of garlic to your cooking. It is a good natural antibiotic and helps keep the bowels regular.

Heart and circulation   Get your protein from fish, millet, poultry and some low-fat dairy products. Use meat infrequently. Have plenty of fibre, as together with strawberries, garlic, olive oil, apples, onions and baked beans, it helps to reduce the cholesterol in your blood. All these, with a reduction of the caffeine and salt that you consume, will also help to keep your blood pressure down. Exercise is absolutely vital. Do what you can, even if it is some form of regular physical exertion in bed or your armchair. Most local authorities run classes and swimming sessions for the older person.

Essential foods

Strawberries   Due to their cleansing and purifying action, they are a great help for all the joint diseases.

Turnips   They are powerful eliminators of uric acid, so help gout and other joint problems. They are useful for the treatment of chest infections – puréed in a little milk is the traditional European folk remedy for bronchitis.

Millet   Rich in protein and low in starch, it is easy to digest and does not cause wind. It contains silicon which is needed for the skin, hair, nails and for the health of the walls of blood vessels.

217

Dried fruits   A superb source of energy, fibre, vitamin A (apricots, peaches and nectarines), dates and figs are good sources of iron and calcium.

Pears   There is some vitamin C in the skin, and if ripe, lots of fruit sugar for rapid energy. They are rich in potassium, which is important if you are taking diuretic pills (water tablets).

Chicken   This is a great form of low-fat protein which is good value.

Chicory   It stimulates the gall bladder to produce bile, which makes it an aid to liver function and digestion.

Garlic   This has to be the great grand-daddy of all the food plants which have therapeutic properties. No matter what you may think about the smell, put it into savoury dishes each day, and if you get a cold, you can even eat it on toast.

Back to basics

Almost everyone will suffer some degree of back pain at some time in their life. Many of these attacks will be mild, many more severe and some excruciating and disabling. After one episode of acute back ache you are 50 per cent more likely to have another one than you were to have the first. The effects of back ache are widespread. Social, economic and medical factors are involved. A bad back stops you enjoying life, playing sports, going dancing, mowing the lawn or even just walking the dog. Thirty-five million working days are lost each year in this country just through the problems of back ache. Personal finances are affected too, as is the whole of industry through lost productivity.

The purpose of these exercises is to help you help yourself to a better back. Even if you've never had a serious problem, the exercises are important. If you have suffered from episodes of back pain they are vital, since maintaining the strength and suppleness of the muscles and ligaments together with the maximum mobility of the spinal joints is the key to prevention, and prevention is better than cure. If you are having any sort of treatment for back pain do speak to your medical practitioner or your osteopath before you start any form of exercises.

Any sports coach, or music teacher for that matter, will tell you that practice makes perfect. There is no point in having a one hour lesson once a week and ignoring the good advice and instruction for the remaining six days and twenty-three hours. You have to carry the lessons you have learned over into your normal life and make a supreme effort to incorporate them into your everyday patterns of work, rest and play. Your body has developed its own habits of posture and muscle tone and to overcome the handicaps you will have to make yourself constantly aware of how you sit, stand, move, work and exercise. By your own effort of consciousness you will and can superimpose new, good habits over the old bad ones. If you do this enough, the new patterns will become the normal ones for your body.

Posture is a full-time function and must be correctly maintained during every waking hour. Posture is also an outward portrayal of inner emotions and again the vicious circle of pain, inactivity, pain and depression is a vital contributor to any back problem. You can put these problems out of your mind right now. No, that's no idle promise but a guarantee. Most back sufferers, you included, can look forward to years of active living. You will have occasional episodes but you know how to cope with those. It won't be easy, since you have to work, work and work again at making the postural changes you need. If you have the commitment and the self-discipline, you will make these changes. The leopard will always change his spots, and even the oldest dog can learn new tricks if the rewards are tempting enough. Your reward will be many years of happy fulfilment in terms of pain-free exercise and activity.

The following exercises should be done for one minute every day and you will soon develop a new strength and mobility in your back which you never dreamed was possible. For those of you who are back sufferers, before you start any of the other exercises, you should concentrate on the following fundamentals in order to relieve the pain of acute episodes and to get things moving once again.

Let's start with a low back stretching and postural exercise. Acute or chronic pain, injury, stress and muscle spasm can be the last straw that initiates the vicious circle by which a trigger point of fibrous tissue is created. This causes continual irritation which in turn causes more pain and more muscle contraction. The following stretching exercises are designed to lengthen both muscles and ligaments, thereby breaking into the cycle and changing the established patterns of the tissues involved. Before starting the exercises, you may find that applications of ice packs (frozen peas are ideal), gentle heat, or the alternate use of both, will induce relaxation of the tissues and make things just a little more comfortable. It makes the movements easier and will remove the acute back pain.

First let's start with flexion of the lower back. Use the legs as a lever to flex the lower part of the back. The incorrect grip only overstrains the knee joints without bending the back. This exercise must be done on the floor or on a really firm surface. Bed is not the ideal place. All lying exercises are best performed on the floor, preferably on a thin foam mat; a camping mattress or a sunbed cover is ideal. It also prevents pressure and bruising to the bony areas of the spine and the sancromum. Lie flat with a small cushion under your head. Bend your knees and put your feet flat on the floor. Place your hands behind your thighs just below the knees and using just the arm muscles pull your knees gently towards your head and raise the head up. The pelvis must be raised off the floor. When you reach the limit of movement and comfort hold the position for fifteen seconds. Then try to increase the bend very gently by pulling with the arm muscles. Do this in progressive steps for one minute. So, with your hands behind your knees, raise your head and pull your knees gently towards your chest. Hold them in that position –

Lower back flexion

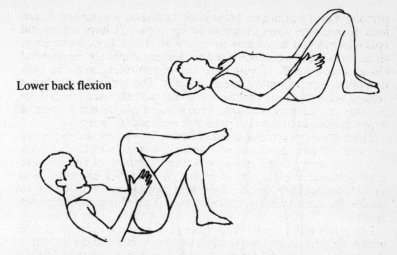

that's very good – quite still – don't stop breathing – hold them where they are – and very gently relax your arms and let your feet go back to the floor.

Let's do it again. Raise your head and pull the knees gently towards your chest; perhaps you can pull them just a little bit further this time. Hold the position where they are, hold them, and gently let the feet go back to the floor. Now for the third time, let's try and get those bones just a little bit further up. Raise the head, bend your arms and pull the knees towards the chest. Pull a little harder; if it doesn't hurt you can pull just a little bit further. Each time you do it you should be able to get your knees a fraction closer to your chest.

Relax and let's do it just one more time. Raise the head, bring the arms up and pull the knees towards the chest. Get them right up. The muscles should be stretching nicely and you should be able to hold your knees almost on to your chest. Very good. Let's go to the next exercise now.

Before we go on to the next exercise, it's very important to lower your legs flat on to the floor one at a time. Holding your right leg with your right hand, release the left leg and straighten it very gently. Now, straighten the other leg. This avoids the possibility of pain caused by a sudden return of both legs to the floor together.

Now let's move on to the side-bending exercise. You should stand up for this one. This exercise will help to stretch the low back and shoulder muscles. Stand with your feet about 18 inches apart and with a very slow and deliberate movement let's just bend to the left, pushing your left hand down the outside of your left thigh towards your knee. Very gently, don't let yourself bend forwards or

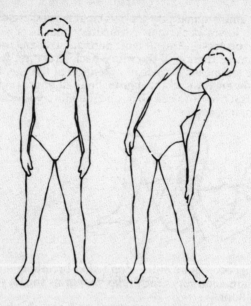

Side bend

backwards. Hold that position – that's very good. Slowly up to the straight position, and let's bend to the right. Gently down as far as you can without causing any pain and remember, don't bend forward. Slowly up again, and let's go down to the left for the second time.

Hold that position for a couple of seconds, gently up and down to the right. Try to push that hand just a little further down towards your knee. Gently up again and to the left – a little bit further this time, right down towards the knee and up and to the right. No bending forward, no bending backward – hold the position and gently up again.

As you find these bends easier, you can bend the knee on the side to which you are moving. Let's just try that. Bend gently to the left, bend the left knee. Don't bend forward. This will enable you to stretch the spinal muscles just a little bit further, and up straight, and slowly to the right, bending the right knee as well. That's much better, you can almost reach the knee now. Okay, let's move on to the important exercise of keeping your back as flat as possible.

An exaggerated inward curve at the base of the spine which makes the buttocks stick out is very common. This excessive curve distorts the entire spinal posture and creates pressure on the rear parts of the lower back joints, squeezing the discs and putting pressure on the nerves, encouraging permanent changes in muscles and the ligament tension of the whole back structure. Learning to tuck in your tail means a constant repetition of the exercises and a concentration on your posture throughout all your waking hours. It's jolly difficult but you can do it, and the more you practise it the more natural it becomes.

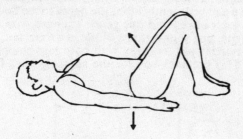

Pelvic tilt (a)

So we are going to do the tail-tucking exercise, starting with the pelvic tilt. This is a very good exercise for all types of back pain, even acute disc pains. It's much easier to do it lying on the floor. So, let's have you on the floor, on your nice foam mattress, flat on your back with both knees bent and your feet flat on the floor. For comfort put a small pillow under your head. The first stage is to press the small of your back down onto the floor, flattening the curve of your lumbar spine. Practise this by putting one hand on the floor under your back and feeling the downward pressure on the hand as you contract your tummy and buttock muscles, both at the same time. If you've got it right you'll feel a slight squeezing sensation in the hip and thigh muscles. Once you've mastered the knack of flattening your back you can move on to raising your buttocks off the floor. You must not lift your back from the ground. This produces the old-fashioned wrestler's bridge position and that increases the curved position. You have to use your abdominal and thigh muscles in this movement.

Let's try it. Knees bent, feet flat on the ground and try to flatten the hollow part of your back against the floor. That's fine. Now, keeping your back in that position try to raise your hips off the floor by pressing with your thigh and buttock muscles. Don't arch your back – hold it in that lifted position and relax. Once you've got the hang of that movement you can do a nice gentle rhythmic pelvic movement – flatten your back, raise the pelvis and hold it for a few seconds, just like that – but don't move yet. Now relax the pelvis, but make sure that you keep your back as we had it. Rest for a couple of seconds, take a deep breath, let yourself relax. Make sure you've kept your hollow back flat against the floor and raise the pelvis, hold it for a few seconds, and relax again. Now raise the pelvis again. We've got a nice gentle and rhythmic movement of raising the pelvis up and down. Let's lift it up, and relax back onto the floor. And once more, lift up, and relax. And let's do it for a last time, lift the pelvis, keeping the back flat, hold it in that position, don't let it curve and very gently lower the pelvis to the floor again.

Now, once you've mastered this gentle exercise, you can start gradually straightening your legs just a little at a time, until you can do the same exercise just as easily with both legs straight out in front of you. This prepares you for the standing back-flattening exercise.

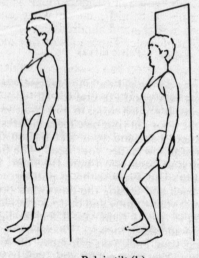

Pelvic tilt (b)

Let's have you standing up with your back against the wall. Right, let's put the feet about 6 inches away from the wall, press the small of your back against the wall and slowly move your buttocks off the wall, keeping your lower back in constant contact with it. Now, very slowly bend the knees, keeping your low back firmly pressed against the wall and your tail well tucked in. This simple procedure strengthens the really big muscles in the front of the thigh (very important for proper lifting), it teaches you to bend with your tail well and truly tucked in, avoiding the pain and unnecessary stress, and above all it starts to improve your conception of upright posture (see diagram on page 224).

Let's try it again. Press the small of your back against the wall, slowly move your buttocks away from the wall, keeping your back in constant contact with it and slowly bend the knees, straighten the legs and bend the knees again. And straighten, and once more let's bend the knees, sliding down the wall. Hold it in that position and gently straighten the legs and relax.

One of the important factors in posture is learning to stand tall. Posture is a subconscious concept; we don't think about the muscles we use to maintain it, or what they are all doing from minute to minute. Why don't you fall over when you raise one arm to the side? Why don't you pitch face down in the dirt when you bend to weed the garden? How can you stand on one leg? All these are made possible by the endless contraction and relaxation of your postural muscles and you don't know a thing about them. Think of the high-wire man balancing with his pole, making endless minute movements to keep his balance a hundred feet up in the air. Your muscles are just like his pole. Thousands of tiny movements and corrections every minute.

Unfortunately, we develop bad posture or habits very quickly and very easily. They are much more difficult to eradicate than they are to learn, and the best way I have found to learn to stand tall is the old-fashioned deportment trick. Practise standing and walking with a book on your head – and a fairly solid, heavy one at that. The mere fact of pushing up against a heavy balanced weight realigns the body and helps to flatten out exaggerated curves in the neck as well as in the lower back. So let's find a nice heavy book, put it on the head and gently walk around the room for a few seconds.

Now we're ready for some slightly more strenuous exercises. We are going to start with a fairly easy one. I call it 'the penny squeeze'. You need a two pence piece and you need to stand up straight with the two pence piece gripped between the cheeks of your bottom. The exercise is to flatten the lower part of your back. Keeping the coin held firmly in place, walk round and round your room, for about a minute. Off you go, and don't let go of the coin. I know it sounds strange but it's a very effective exercise.

Let's move on now to the head-up exercise. For this let's have us back on the floor again. Knees bent, feet flat on the floor, small cushion under the head. Start by flattening the hollow of the back onto the floor. Raise your arms up above your shoulders. Put your chin on your chest and roll gently forward until the shoulder blades are just off the floor. Don't try to sit up – just roll gently forward. Your back won't be more than an inch or two off the floor. Hold that position. That's right – it's not so difficult. Now roll gently back

Head-up

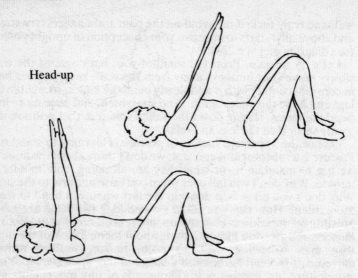

onto the floor, keeping your tail well and truly tucked in. Let's do that ten times. Roll up, and hold it, and down, and 2 and up, and down. And 3, up we go – not too far, keep the tail tucked in, and roll gently back onto the floor. And up again for number 4, hold the position, and roll back. And 5 and back, and 6 and back, and 7 and back, and 8 and I know it's getting more difficult but the more you do it, the easier it'll become. And back, and struggle for number 9, up you come, keep the back flat and relax. And finally number 10, up you go, hold it for a second, and down. Well done. Just rest where you are with the feet flat on the floor and the knees bent and take two or three nice deep breaths.

Everybody's heard of sit-ups – they are bad for people with back problems. What we're going to do is what I call the sit-down.

You must be really proficient at this one before you even consider trying a sit-up. Let's start by sitting on the floor with the knees bent and your arms around your knees. To do this exercise, lean very slowly backward, using your arms to support all the weight of your trunk. Now use your arm muscles to pull yourself back into the sitting position. Just try it, lean back, just move a few inches backward, and pull up with your arms. You see, it's quite easy. Let's do ten of those, and lean back, and pull up with your arms, and back for number two, and pull up with the arms, and 3 and up, and 4 and up, and 5 and up, and 6 and up, and 7, don't forget to use your arms only to pull up, and 8 and up, and 9 and up, and 10 and up again. Have a little rest. As you do this exercise more and more,

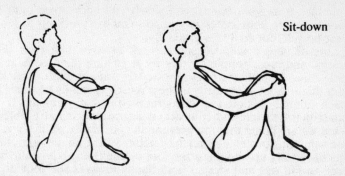

Sit-down

your abdominal muscles will get stronger and stronger so that you will be able to use less pull with the arms and eventually you will be able to go much further back and come up without even using your arms at all. When you can do that ten times without feeling any discomfort, then and only then can you go on and do the sit-up.

Sit-up

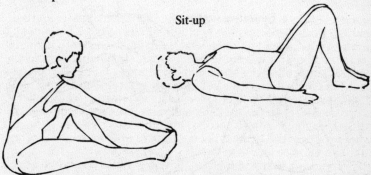

The same position, flat on the back, knees bent, feet flat on the floor. Tuck in the tail, push your chin down on to your chest, your hands by your sides. Now I want you to roll yourself slowly upright from the neck, keeping your tail tucked in. Up you come, roll forward. Once you're up you can straighten your legs to the floor and stretch your fingers forward to the toes. Now roll slowly back onto the floor, bending your knees back up again as you go. Let's try it. Tuck in the tail, put the chin on the chest, and roll slowly upright. As you get there, straighten your legs and stretch forward with your fingers towards your toes. Roll slowly down and bend your knees. Let's try one more of those. Chin on chest, roll slowly upward from the neck, straighten the legs, stretch forward towards your toes from your hands, and slowly roll back down onto the floor, bending your knees as you go. You can work up to ten of these as well, but do it very gradually.

Lots of people who do sports work at stretching their hamstrings, and most people do that by stretching them both at the same time. Your hamstrings are the large muscles at the back of your thigh. A lot of elasticity in these muscles actually prevents too much lumbar flexion and encourages spinal movement. If the hamstrings shorten and contract, it aggravates spinal problems. What we are going to do to prevent any possibility of injury is the one hamstring protected stretch exercise. Sitting on the floor, bend one knee fully up and place the foot on the floor. Allow the bent knee to fall out and stretch both hands towards the foot of the straight leg as far as is comfortable. Now, let's start a gentle, rhythmical, bouncing movement reaching towards the foot. Try it for twenty seconds. Very good. Bounce yourself gently up and down, sit up straight and rest. Now let's change legs. Bend the other knee, place the other foot flat on the floor. Let the bent knee fall

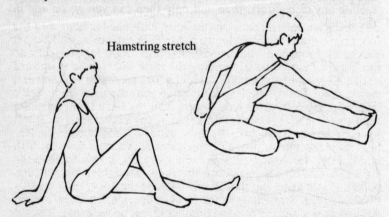

Hamstring stretch

outward and stretch both hands towards the foot of the straight leg as far as you can. Bounce up and down very gently for twenty seconds. Let's change legs again, and repeat it both sides. Are you bouncing towards the leg? Very good, make sure that the bent leg falls out as far as you can. This protects that hamstring from being overstretched. Then let's change legs once more, let the leg fall out and stretch towards the straightened foot, and bounce gently up and down. Very good, straighten both legs, flat on the back, take a deep breath in . . . and right out . . . and relax.

Let's go on to the leg-lifting exercises now. Lifting the weight of both legs off the floor together puts a really severe strain on the

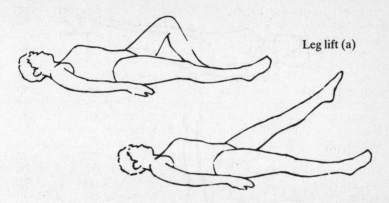

Leg lift (a)

lower back joints, and unless you already have superb muscle control, this will inevitably increase the curvature in your lower back. This often causes pain. Until you are several weeks into your exercise programme we'll stay with lifting one leg at a time. So, to do the leg up, let's lie back on the floor, with one leg bent with the foot on the floor, the other leg straight. Tuck the tail in, and keep it tucked in throughout the exercise. With the right leg straight and the left leg bent, without bending the right knee, raise it upward until it is level with the left knee. Hold it for a second or two, lower it slowly to the floor. And let's lift it again. Lift the right leg until it's level with the left knee. And lower. And the third time, raise the right leg, don't let it bend, don't raise it any higher than your left knee, and lower it slowly to the floor. And once more, raise the leg, hold it for a second or two, and slowly down. And let's have the fifth and last one, raise the right leg, keep it straight, no higher than the left knee, and slowly back onto the floor. Straighten the left leg, bend the right knee, put the right foot flat on the floor, and now let's lift the left leg. Straight up to the level of the right knee, and relax. And lift again, and down. And number three, up we come, lower it very gently. Number four, lift up, don't bend the left knee, keep the left leg straight, don't lift it higher than the right knee, and slowly down. And the fifth and last one, slowly up, hold the leg straight, and lower gently to the floor.

When you've done the exercises for a few weeks, and you've really got the muscles working much better and much stronger than they were, we can start lifting both legs together. Now, for this exercise, you do not start with both feet on the floor. Let's have you lying flat on the floor with your heels resting on the seat of an armchair. Your legs should be at an angle of about 30°. By starting in this position you are avoiding using a muscle called the iliopsoas. This increases your lumbar curve. So, to do the exercise, tuck the

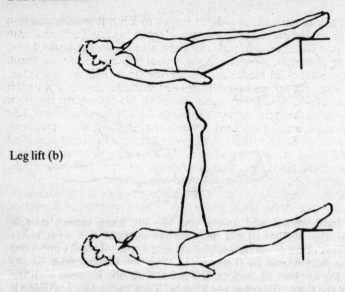

Leg lift (b)

tail in, maintain it in this position throughout the exercise, and, keeping both knees straight, raise the legs to 90°, up you come, and lower them slowly. Rest for a second or two, and raise them again. And slowly down back onto the chair. And let's just try a third one. Lift up, and slowly down. You should be able to build up to at least ten repetitions of this exercise, but not yet. You do it very gradually, and you only increase by another one or two at a time as long as they don't hurt.

Now, we're going to do what I call the crossover sit-up. In this exercise we lie flat on the back with both legs straight out in front of

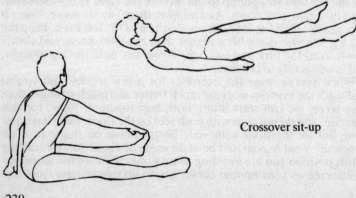

Crossover sit-up

you. Tuck in the tail, and don't forget to keep it in that position throughout the exercise. Spread your legs 45° apart. Tuck your chin down into the chest and put your right arm across the body. Now, pushing your right shoulder towards your left leg, raise your trunk until both shoulder blades are just off the floor. Lift up, and relax. And again, lift up, and push your right shoulder towards your left leg, and down. And lift up again, shoulder blades just off the floor and pushing the right shoulder towards the left leg and down. And the last time, and lift up, push towards the left foot, and relax. Now change arms. Stretch the left shoulder towards the right leg. And up, and down, and up, and down. And lift up, get those shoulder blades off the floor, and stretch towards the foot, and down. And number four, lift up, and down. And relax.

You must build up to a ten-minute routine of these exercises. They must be done every single day. Three months of dedicated work will do wonders for your back. You may enjoy raising the level of your back fitness in many ways, but a large number of people find that sport is an important factor in getting and keeping fit. Since you already have a back problem, there are some sports which are not the most suitable. You may make a conscious decision to suffer some discomfort in order to enjoy your favourite sport. After all, hurt is not always the same as harm, and provided that you are not in an acute stage of severe back pain, you would be better off enjoying an important cricket match, a round of golf, or a game of badminton, and being uncomfortable for a few days afterwards, rather than staying at home getting more and more depressed about all the fun you are missing. I do advise my back patients to avoid weight-lifting, judo, rowing, violent squash and all contact sports, especially rugby, and above all, jogging, since your feet will hit the ground with all your body weight – around one thousand times for every mile. Swimming, preferably not the breast stroke, cycling, walking, ice or roller skating, are all suitable forms of exercise. But, do be sensible, and, above all, care for your back, no one else can.

Risk and stress

'The ultimate measure of a man is not where he stands in moments of comfort and convenience, but where he stands at times of challenge and controversy.' So said Martin Luther King.

At moments of comfort and convenience stress is not a problem, but when challenge and controversy stare us in the face, the way in which we react, physically, emotionally and spiritually, is the measure of our success in dealing with stress. Stress is part of everyday life, and our bodies' responses to stressful stimuli have always played a key role in mankind's survival.

The 'fight or flight' response which prepares our bodies for instant reaction at times of danger, and which our bodies produce without conscious effort or command, is the root cause of all the problems associated with our inability to cope with the stresses produced in industrialised Western civilisation. This remarkable ability to react instantly to challenge becomes counterproductive when it is impossible to choose either 'fight' or 'flight', when the only option is to 'grin and bear it' or 'grit our teeth' or 'soldier on' – all expressions which betray the emotions. Many people are ill-equipped to deal with excessive stresses, and stress-induced illness is growing to epidemic proportions. Heart attack, high blood pressure, insomnia, premenstrual tension, menopausal problems, sexual disorders, skin complaints, digestive and bowel disturbances, asthma, migraine and arthritis can all be directly linked to, or caused by, poor coping with stress.

The idea that stress-related disasters are the exclusive province of the boardroom and high-powered executive is just not true. No one is immune from this plague. It exists on the factory floor, in the typing pool, at the kitchen sink, in the elderly and the young alike.

While attitudes to the over-stressed patient are thankfully, beginning to change, the orthodox medical approach frequently fails to recognise or deal with the root of the problem. The symptoms are treated, but seldom the patient. The physician may not recognise the effects that the patient's mental state is having on his or her body. The psychiatrist may well ignore physical disease altogether. The epidemic of stress disorders is only equalled by the pandemic of prescriptions for anti-depressant and tranquillising drugs – and the consequent dependence on these by millions of people.

Sweeping the dirt of stress under the pharmacological carpet of behaviour-modifying drugs is not a solution. There is no better example of the need for a holistic approach to health than in this field. Nor is there a single answer to dealing with the vast range of problems produced by stress. The most important steps that any of us take along the road to coping with it are to recognise it, understand it, use 'good' stress to our advantage, deal with 'bad' stress and cope with the stresses of family, work, social and environmental situations.

After thirty years in practice it would be all too easy to hurry patients through my consulting rooms using the 'pill for every ill' approach. After all, writing the prescription is the quickest way of terminating the consultation. This attitude would surely solve my problems and relieve much of my stress, but in the long term it just doesn't work. The only real help when stress becomes a problem is self-help.

First know thine enemy

The original engineering definition of stress is 'a force which acts on a body, setting up strains within it according to its load-carrying capacity, flexibility and tolerance'. When the force exerted exceeds the tolerance of a particular body, something has to give, and the human body is no different.

Individuals vary enormously in ability to withstand stress. Some can take as much in one hour as would lay low others if it were spread over a year. Many 'high-flyers' seem to not only thrive on it, but to need it as a constant spur. Frequently this type of person is, in reality, addicted to his or her own stress and the continual outpouring of adrenalin which it produces.

Whatever you may think your threshold of tolerance is, you can be certain that even you have a limit, and it is likely to be lower than your estimate. The risk of stress is that it is insidious. Like the furring up of your water pipes, it is not till the last grain of deposit blocks the flow of water and the pipe bursts that you know about it. So you have to be able to recognise how much you as an individual can tolerate, and how to take the appropriate steps to deal with this silent, stealthy and ruthless enemy.

Are you stressed?

It is often difficult to take an objective view of yourself to see if how you feel is related to external factors. Some common signs of stress are easy to spot. Ask yourself if you:

- Feel near to tears much of the time.
- Fidget, bite your nails or fiddle with your hair.

- Find it hard to concentrate, and impossible to make decisions.
- Find it increasingly hard to talk to people.
- Snap and shout at those around you at home and work.
- Eat when you're not hungry.
- Feel tired much of the time.
- Think that your sense of humour has gone for good.
- Feel suspicious of others.
- No longer have any interest in sex.
- Sleep badly.
- Drink and/or smoke more to help you through those difficult days.
- Ever feel that you just can't cope.

If you answer *yes* to more than four of these questions, you are stressed. *Do something!* You cannot carry on as you are.

The As and Bs of stress

It is possible to separate people into two distinct personality types – A and B.

TYPE A

Very competitive
Bossy, forceful
Gets things done quickly (not always well)
Strives for promotion and status
Eager for recognition and fame
Quick tempered
Restless when unoccupied
Speaks quickly and explosively
Moves, walks and eats quickly
Will not put up with delay
Thrives on the pressure of doing several projects at the same time
Likes to be given deadlines and beat them

TYPE B

Uncompetitive
Easygoing and reticent
Slow and methodical
Doesn't care about status or promotion
Shuns the limelight
Slow to anger
Enjoys creative leisure
Speaks slowly
Does not rush at or into anything

Risk and stress

Does not mind delay
Enjoys doing one thing at a time
Ignores deadlines

There is a proven link between behaviour patterns and the susceptibility to coronary heart disease. Type A people, whose lives are full of stressful behaviour, are more likely to succumb than type Bs, who have a more relaxed approach to life. If you identify with the type A pattern and fit half or more of the characteristics, then you are a Type A person. If you want to avoid 'overstress' or a heart attack, try to adjust your lifestyle and take in more of the type B attitudes.

Dealing with stress

Once you have established your 'stress threshold', how do you deal with the stress that you cannot use? Many people can work out their own methods. For some it is a hobby like gardening or painting; for others, the cinema, theatre or music; for many it may be a sport.

In fact, physical exercise is recommended by the experts as a particularly good form of relaxation. It gets rid of pent-up energy and encourages self-confidence. It is worth noting that endurance runners, covering long distances each week, tend to be less anxious and more emotionally stable than their physically less active contemporaries.

De-Stress the distress

If you think that you are unreasonably stressed, you can help yourself to break out of the vicious circle.

* Do not work more than nine hours daily.
* Take at least half an hour off in the day.
* Take at least one and a half days out of your normal working routine each week.
* Eat regular and healthy meals.
* Get regular exercise.
* Practise some form of relaxation technique.
* Face up to work or relationship problems and do something to resolve them.
* Do not use alcohol, caffeine, nicotine or drugs to relieve stress.
* Remember that stressful situations are not always the unhappy ones.
* Getting married, promoted or moving house all cause stress.
* Learn to recognise your own thresholds.
* Use stress positively and channel your energy into making your life better.

236

Stress can be good for you

You can't spend your life avoiding stress, and you should not try to. For lots of people it is enjoyable to use their stress to overcome physical, intellectual and social challenges. Extending yourself in this way keeps you healthy, active and young – as long as you also have the ability to relax. By learning to face each new challenge as it comes along, and by knowing how to switch off before fatigue and exhaustion set in, you can use your stress to make life more interesting, exciting and fulfilling.

That's what takes the risk out of stress.

Relaxacise

You can't open a newspaper, read a magazine, or turn on the radio today, without hearing something about stress. And most of it is pretty bad. Not all stress, however, is bad. Our responses to stress are what have enabled us to survive as a species. Where we get into trouble is when we can't respond in the proper way to stress. The well-known fright, fight and flight syndrome is the key to the entire problem. When man is exposed to some sort of unpleasant stimulus, his body reacts by producing vast quantities of a chemical called adrenalin, and this prepares us either to run away or to fight back. And in today's modern society we are constantly subjected to a bombardment of stimuli and nearly always are unable to act in the appropriate way. If you have a disagreement with your boss at work, you can't run away, and you can't fight back. If you work in a shop and you are dealing with a difficult customer, you have to grit your teeth and grin and bear it.

This is the sort of stress which creates problems, because all this unused adrenalin builds up in the system, causing muscle tension, making the blood pressure go up and creating all the possible problems of these two effects: aches and pains, high blood pressure, which can result in heart disease, or a stroke. And all sorts of debilitating problems, such as migraine, skin diseases, asthma, even some other allergies, are directly linked to excessive stress. The aim here is not in any way to teach people to avoid stress, because stress in our modern society, for most of us, cannot possibly be avoided. The idea is to teach you how to cope with stress in a simple, safe and very easy manner.

One of the commonest side effects of stress is muscle tension. The body very quickly adapts to new patterns of muscle tone and what for a small child would be unbearably uncomfortable, for the adult subjected to repetitive stresses becomes the norm. You get used to your own body's stresses and in fact there are many people who get addicted to stress. The typical example of the weekend migraine used to be the preserve of busy executive businessmen, but with more and more women taking on high-powered and demanding jobs, it's just as common with businesswomen too. You struggle through the week coping with problems, with excesses, with difficulties. The minute you get home on Friday evening and unwind, the migraine starts. A stress reaction.

What I am going to do is to teach you how to teach your body to reawaken its awareness of relaxation and to be more aware of the discomforts of muscular stress and strain. The easiest way to achieve this is by recreating muscle fatigue. The important thing is to give yourself time – allow yourself half an hour at the end of the day. Make yourself comfortable. These exercises are best done lying flat on the floor, on a nice thick rug or a thin foam mattress, the sort of thing you have on a sun lounger, or for camping. Wrap yourself in a light, thin but warm blanket, take the telephone off the hook, lock the door, draw the blinds, and shut yourself away from the demands of the outside world. And this includes husbands, wives, parents, children, neighbours – shut them all out and give yourself half an hour to relearn the natural way of coping with stress.

What we're going to do is to take your body through a series of muscle contractions and relaxations, exerting those muscles in such a way that at the end of the series of exercises the muscles will be suffering fatigue. The result of this fatigue is complete and total relaxation. So, are you lying flat on the floor, comfortably with a small pillow under your head, with loose comfortable clothing, and warm? Let's begin.

I want you to close your eyes, and I want you to start by stretching your left leg as hard as you can away from your body. Push it down, keeping it in contact with the floor, pointing your toes and contracting all the muscles of the calf and thigh and pointing your toes down as hard as you can. Really push, don't let go yet, keep holding on to those muscles. And relax. Now let's do the same thing with the right leg. Push that leg straight down along the floor away from your trunk, point the toes down, contract the calf muscles and really squeeze the muscles of your thigh. Push hard, don't let go yet, keep pushing. Keep pushing with that leg, and relax. Now let's push both legs together, push down as hard as you can. Push those legs away from your trunk, point the toes down, squeeze the calf muscles, squeeze the thigh muscles, feel your bottom muscles squeezing as hard as you can. Keep pushing, keep pushing – your muscles are probably starting to tremble a little bit now – that's good. Don't let go yet, don't stop breathing. And relax.

Now let's do the same thing with the left arm. I want you to push your left arm as hard as you can down along the side of your body. Push the hand towards the feet, spread your fingers as wide as you can. Press down with the shoulder muscles, contract the arm muscles, contract the shoulder muscles. Push as hard as you can. Don't let go yet – keep pushing, keep pushing. And relax. Now let's do the same thing with the right arm. Push the arm as hard as you can along your side towards your right foot. Spread the fingers as wide as possible, feel the muscles of the forearm contracting. Press with the shoulder, keep pressing, keep breathing. You don't have to stop breathing. Keep pressing with that arm. And relax. Now let's press both arms. Stretch them down from the shoulders, stretch hard, spread the fingers as wide as you can. Feel those forearm muscles contracting, feel your biceps and your triceps, keep pressing, spread the fingers, spread the fingers. Are your muscles trembling? You're doing it right. Keep pressing, and relax.

Now, we're going to press everything together. I want you to stretch your legs and arms as hard as you can, and push. Stretch the legs down, push the arms down, with your hands reaching towards your feet. Point the toes down, contract the calf muscles, squeeze the bottom muscles, push with the shoulders, spread the fingers as wide as possible. Hold it all like that, but do keep breathing. Push a little harder, wait for those muscles to start trembling. Keep pushing, don't give up yet, just a little bit harder. And relax. Take a very deep breath in. Breathe in . . . fill your lungs, expand your chest as far as you can, and push the breath out. And breathe in again, as far as you can, a little bit more, stretch your rib cage, hold your breath, and push it out. One more deep, deep breath. Breathe in . . . hold your breath . . . and breathe out. Now we'll do it all again.

Let's start with the left leg. Stretch your left leg down from your trunk, point the toe, squeeze the calf muscle, contract the thigh muscles, and push. Keep holding it, push as hard as you can. Keep pushing, keep pushing. And relax the leg. Now the right leg. Push, push, push, point the toe, squeeze the calf muscles, squeeze the thigh muscles. Feel that leg really begin to tremble now. Keep pushing, keep pushing, hold it still, don't stop breathing. And relax the leg. Now let's do both legs together. And push as hard as you can. Point the toes down, squeeze the calf muscles, feel your buttock muscles squeezing as hard as they possibly can. Push with the thigh muscles, keep pushing with those legs, keep breathing, and push, and push, and make those legs tremble with the effort of using the muscles. Keep pushing, and relax.

Now the left arm, push down from the shoulder, stretch the fingers as wide as you can, push the hand towards the left foot. Feel those shoulder muscles, feel the muscles in your forearm, hold them steady, hold it, don't let go yet. Keep pushing, keep pushing, and relax. And now, the right arm. Push down, stretch the fingers, push from the shoulder, feel those forearm muscles, feel the arm beginning to tremble. Keep breathing, keep breathing, don't let go of that arm yet. Keep pushing, and relax. Now both arms again, push down, stretch the fingers as far as possible, feel the shoulders pushing down, feel the forearm muscles, push with the biceps, push with the triceps. Hold both arms, keep pushing, keep pushing – if those arms aren't trembling you aren't pushing hard enough. Keep pushing and keep breathing. Hold it, hold it steady. And relax again.

Now, let's have both arms and both legs together, and a big, big push with everything. Push with the arms, push with the shoulders, spread those fingers a little wider. Point those toes down as far as you can. Feel the buttock muscles contracting, squeeze the calves, push with the thigh muscles, spread the fingers. Hold everything just like that and push just as hard as you can. Don't stop breathing, keep pushing, keep pushing, keep pushing hard – everything should be trembling nicely. Keep pushing, and relax again.

Take a deep, deep breath in, breathe in . . . fill those lungs up, expand your chest, and push the breath out. And another deep breath in . . . right in, as far as you can, and just a little bit further, push that oxygen into your lungs, and breathe right out . . . . And one more really deep, deep breath, breathe in . . . a little bit more, a little bit more, hold your breath, and very slowly let the breath out as gently as you can . . . right out . . . right out. And just rest where you are for a moment.

Doesn't that feel good? All the tensions just wash away. The stresses of the day are breathed out with your last slow breath. As with any form of exercise, if you are really going to benefit from these simple relaxation techniques, you really have to practise.

It can be helpful to do these exercises to suitable music. While you're listening you can do the same sequence another three times. Don't forget, it's left leg, right leg, both legs together, left arm, right arm, both arms together, and then arms and legs at the same time. Don't forget to breathe while you're pushing, and don't forget to take three really deep breaths in and out between each group of exercises. The more you practise, the easier it becomes. When you've done five sequences of this exercise you will feel beautifully and peacefully relaxed. In time you will be able to achieve the same degree of relaxation with just one sequence of exercises, or maybe with just the very thought of relaxation.

The four seasons

Throughout this book you will find helpful information which is useful during the year and will help keep you and your family healthy. But, just as the seasons change so there are special health needs created by climatic conditions and seasonal activities. In this chapter you will find advice on spring cleaning your system, coping with summer problems, weathering the winter ills and surviving the rigours of Christmas.

I apologise in advance for some small duplications of information given elsewhere in the book, but by putting the facts all together in this section you'll find all you need to know easily accessible and at your fingertips.

At the end of this section there is a three-week healthy weight loss plan which is suitable for any time of the year, and can be adapted to include fresh produce that is available when you decide to try the diet. Wherever possible use fruits, salads and vegetables which are fresh and in season.

Spring clean diet

Twenty years ago I met a remarkable Swiss man called Fred Pestalozzi. Fred is the owner of a laboratory high in the hills over-looking Lake Zurich, where Bio-Strath is made. This vigorous and dedicated man made a lasting impression on me as being one of the very few people working in the field of herbal medicine who was using the scientific methods of today together with the ancient ideas of the traditional herbalists. We have been friends and colleagues ever since, and it is his research that led to the 'Bio-Strath 7-Day Diet'.

Realising that so many people paid little attention to their diet for most of the time, Fred Pestalozzi decided to produce a really healthy, safe and effective 'spring clean' regime. With typical Swiss thoroughness he spent two years experimenting, with the help of Dr Sabine Grieder of the world-famous Bircher Benner clinic in Zurich. The final diet was tested on 300 members of the readers' panel of the Swiss magazine *Elle*.

The results were exciting. Not only did most people lose between 3 and 8 lb, but 260 out of the 300 in the experiment said they felt an improvement in their general state of health and well-being that was 'good' or 'excellent'.

The four seasons

So now, here's your chance to give your whole system a thorough 'spring clean' and lose a few pounds at the same time, as well as feeling really great after just seven days of healthy eating.

Most people just can't eat all the food that is allowed, and except for the first day of the diet, you will not even feel hungry. Bio-Strath, a natural food supplement made from yeast, wild herbs, honey and pure orange juice, is a great aid to dieting. It helps the metabolism, stops you feeling tired, and promotes a general improvement in well-being and natural resistance. You should take two 5 ml teaspoons of Bio-Strath Elixir before each meal.

Since day one is the most severe, it helps to start the diet on a day when you can take things a bit more gently than usual – a Saturday or Sunday suits most people.

First Day
  Breakfast: 2 teaspoons of Bio-Strath, 1 glass of fruit or vegetable juice, 1 portion of natural yoghurt
  Lunch: 2 teaspoons of Bio-Strath, 1 glass of fruit juice and 1 glass of vegetable juice, 1 portion of yoghurt
  Supper: 2 teaspoons of Bio-Strath, 1 glass of fruit or vegetable juice, 1 portion of yoghurt, 1 cup of herb tea (e.g. solidago) or weak Indian tea without sugar

Second Day
  Breakfast: Standard Breakfast consisting of: 2 teaspoons of Bio-Strath, 1 fruit, 1 to 2 slices of wholemeal bread with cottage cheese, 1 portion of yoghurt, 1 cup of weak tea or skimmed milk
  Lunch: 2 teaspoons of Bio-Strath, 1 fruit, about 7 ounces of raw vegetable salad, about 10 ounces of steamed vegetables with one spoon of sunflower oil
  Supper: 2 teaspoons of Bio-Strath, 1 fruit, 5 ounces of muesli mixed with yoghurt, 1 cup of weak tea

Third Day
  Breakfast: Standard Breakfast (as on second day)
  Lunch: 2 teaspoons of Bio-Strath, 1 fruit, 7 ounces of mixed salad, 1 jacket potato with about 2 ounces of cottage cheese with herbs
  Supper: 2 teaspoons of Bio-Strath, 1 portion of yoghurt with fruit added, 1 slice of wholemeal bread with low-fat cheese, 1 cup of weak tea

Fourth day – Rice day
  The total quantity of rice for the day should be prepared in the morning (3 ounces of dry rice cooked in quarter of a pint of

242

water or vegetable broth will produce 7 to 8 ounces)
  Breakfast: 2 teaspoons of Bio-Strath, 5 ounces of boiled rice,
    5 ounces of stewed apple sweetened with honey and
    flavoured with cinnamon and grated lemon rind
  Lunch: 2 teaspoons of Bio-Strath, about 7 ounces of boiled rice,
    7 ounces of steamed vegetables (tomatoes, celery, etc.)
  Supper: 2 teaspoons of Bio-Strath, 5 ounces of boiled rice,
    5 ounces of orange (fleshy part only)

Fifth Day
  Breakfast: Standard Breakfast (as on second and third days)
  Lunch: 2 teaspoons of Bio-Strath, 1 fruit, about 7 ounces of raw
    vegetable salad, 1 jacket potato, about 3 ounces of
    steamed spinach without sauce but mixed with one
    tablespoon of sunflower oil
  Supper: 2 teaspoons of Bio-Strath, 5 ounces of cottage cheese
    mixed to a cream with sour milk and poured over chopped
    fruit, 1 cup of weak tea

Sixth Day
  Breakfast: Standard Breakfast (as on second, third and fifth days)
  Lunch: 2 teaspoons of Bio-Strath, 1 fruit, 7 ounces of mixed
    salad, 1 jacket potato, about 3 ounces of steamed beans
    with 1 tablespoonful of sunflower oil
  Supper: 2 teaspoons of Bio-Strath, 1 fruit, 5 ounces of muesli
    mixed with yoghurt, 1 to 2 slices of wholemeal bread with
    low-fat cheese, 1 cup of weak tea

Seventh Day
  Breakfast: Standard Breakfast (as on second, third, fifth and
    sixth days)
  Lunch: 2 teaspoons of Bio-Strath, 1 fruit, 7 ounces of mixed
    salad, a choice of: boiled potatoes, blue trout (steamed in
    aluminium foil and served with chopped parsley and
    lemon juice) or grilled chopped veal cutlets or vegetarian
    soya cutlet, 1 fruit salad
  Supper: 2 teaspoons of Bio-Strath, 1 fruit and a choice of a lightly
    boiled egg and 1 or 2 slices of wholemeal bread or ham,
    cheese and wholemeal bread (with a little butter), 1 cup of
    weak tea

Well done! You have finished your diet week. You have probably
lost a few pounds and certainly feel great. You can safely repeat this
seven-day diet several times a year and in any case it's a good idea
for the whole family to pick one day out of the diet and stick to it
once a week.

Summer allergies

It's everybody's dream; you wake to the clear blue sky of a summer dawn, the birds are singing, the bees buzzing, the mercury climbing. Thoughts of a long hot day, a picnic in the country and a barbecue in the honeysuckle-scented evening, spur you into action. Or do they?

Not if you are one of the unfortunate 20 per cent of people who suffer from hay fever or asthma, nor if you are amongst the multitude who endure nettle rash, bad reactions to insect bites and stings, sensitivity to sunlight, or any of the allergies which are so prevalent at this time of the year.

If you are amongst the 40 per cent of the population who show a susceptibility to allergy, don't lose heart! There may not be a guaranteed cure for your allergy, but there is a great deal of self-help which can ease your misery, alleviate the worst of the symptoms and let you join in most of the summer fun without spending your days in a darkened room with a crate of kleenex.

All allergies are inappropriate responses by the body's immune system to a substance which is not normally harmful. The immune system is a complex mechanism which helps us combat infections. It does this by identifying 'foreign bodies' and then mobilising the white cells to destroy them. In some people, the system makes mistakes and wrongly identifies an innocent substance as an invader. The white cells over-react, producing large quantities of the chemical, histamine, and the symptoms of asthma, hay fever, eczema and all the other allergies which plague so many people.

Hay fever

Hay fever is an allergy to pollens, specifically from grasses, trees and flowering plants. The symptoms start when the plants are in flower, and the unfortunates who are allergic to many varieties of pollen may suffer from spring to autumn. They have to endure violent bouts of sneezing, itchy and watery eyes, catarrh, blocked sinuses, disturbed sleep and all-round misery. Hay fever is at its worst during hot and windy summer weather.

The same symptoms can be triggered by moulds, feathers, dust, the house dust mite, animal dander – dogs, cats and horses are frequent culprits. If you react to these non-pollen allergens, you have 'perennial rhinitis'. The symptoms are usually less severe, but continue throughout the year.

SELF HELP

There are obvious practical steps which often get ignored:

- Don't go out early in the morning or late in the evening, when pollen counts are high.
- Keep windows closed, especially in the bedroom.
- Don't bring flowers into the house.
- Make someone else mow the lawn.
- Wear glasses or sunspecs when you do go out – they keep the pollen out of your eyes.
- Even if it's hot, keep car windows closed – sweating is better than sneezing.

If you have perennial rhinitis, see Asthma (page 109) for more practical tips on prevention.

Apart from the orthodox anti-allergy drugs, there are natural alternative treatments. An instant way to stop an attack of the sneezes is to sniff cold water up your nose, and spit out through the mouth. I know it sounds disgusting, and the first sniff is, but this simple trick washes all the pollen grains out of the nasal passages. You will be symptom-free till you go out again.

Keep a bottle of distilled water in the fridge, and use it in an eyebath to irrigate the eyes (use clean water for each eye). A used, cold, damp teabag placed over each eye for two minutes, helps stop the irritation.

If you go out when the pollen count is high, use one of the filter masks, available from the chemist – 3M make a very good version, ideal for asthmatics too.

Reducing the amount of dairy products in the diet controls the production of mucus, and makes life more comfortable, though make sure you replace the calcium with a daily supplement like Porosis D, and don't deprive children of milk without professional advice.

New Era combination H is a good homeopathic remedy for hay fever, and 500 mg of vitamin C, taken morning and evening, can help a lot. Inhale with the French essential oil preparation, Climarome, which keeps the nose and sinuses clear. A tablespoon of honey each day is a good old wives' remedy.

Asthma

Not exclusively a summer allergy, it is often much worse at this time of the year. In childhood, asthma is almost always an allergy problem and there is usually some family history. Hay fever and eczema may be present in close relatives and develop in the asthmatic child, together with the breathing difficulties.

There are a number of practical changes which it is vital to implement; these work, too, for perennial rhinitis:

245

● Keep bedrooms cool and draught free, to prevent air currents that waft the dust mite droppings, which are microscopic, into the air, and are then inhaled by the sleeping occupant.
● Avoid furry or hairy pets and cage birds.
● Use smooth, wipeable surfaces in the bedroom. Lino, window blinds, a plastic cover on the mattress, synthetic duvet and pillows, damp dust all surfaces just before bed, vacuum daily with a suction cleaner and include the mattress.
● Always take medication as prescribed by your doctor. Much of it will be for prevention rather than relief of the symptoms and it can be harmful to stop some of the cortisone drugs suddenly.
● Use anti-dust mite carpet shampoo, which works well. Paint for the same purpose is not much good, as the mites live in carpets not on walls!

25 mg of vitamin B6 and 500 mg of C should be taken daily.

Acupuncture often helps, and osteopathic treatment can improve the movement of ribs. Gentle massage to the back is soothing during an attack.

Asthma is a serious disease, sometimes fatal, so if in doubt, *call your doctor*. This condition is a prime example of how some of the unorthodox therapies can be used as complementary medicine, side by side with existing treatment, *not as an alternative to it*.

Things that bite

Wasps are one of the summer terrors. Twenty or so people die each year from their stings, around half due to allergic shock, the rest by asphyxiation after being stung in the mouth or throat. If you are stung, mix a paste of vinegar and salt, to rub into the sting. Bee stings should be removed with tweezers – they are left in the skin – then bathed with a teaspoon of bicarbonate of soda in half a glass of water. If you have a serious reaction to these, ask your GP about a syringe of adrenalin for emergencies.

N.B. Rush to the nearest hospital if there is any difficulty with breathing, swelling away from the site of the sting, blue skin or lips, a sudden flush or rash, a very fast pulse or if the person passes out.

The more you are bitten by mosquitoes, the worse the reaction, so if you come up in great red, itchy lumps, you should take all the preventative action you can. Keep covered up, sleeves rolled down and trousers tucked into socks. Use a good insect repellent: if they get close enough to see you – about one inch – they'll bite.

Another hot summer will produce an even worse plague of cat fleas than last year. The more you get bitten, the stronger the allergic reaction. Buy some flea powder and use regularly.

Special candles that deter insects are OK indoors but not much use in the garden. Two aromatherapy products from the French company, Dr Valnet, are useful. If you are bitten or stung, apply a few drops of Tegarome, a mixture of oils, including lavender, neroli and rosemary. Volarome is a good repellent, particularly against mosquitoes, and includes geranium, mint and sage oils.

Eat plenty of garlic – the bugs don't like the smell.

You can even be allergic to the sun

After the long and gloomy winter, at the first sign of sun, out you rush. Use a good, high-factor sun screen to start with. Never sunbathe between noon and 3 o'clock, don't lie out for more than fifteen minutes at a time for the first few days, replace sun cream often, wear a hat with a good brim, and if you are going topless or wearing a G-string, watch out as breasts and buttocks are not often exposed to the sun, so are much more sensitive.

If you come up in a spotty irritating rash after sunbathing, don't blame your suntan lotion. It is not prickly heat, but more likely to be Polymorphic Light Eruption, an allergy to the sunshine. Cover up for a few days, use a higher factor lotion, and take great care.

Take a daily dose of beta-carotene which your body turns into vitamin A, as added protection for sensitive skin.

Beware the berries

Sadly, some of the things we most look forward to eating during the summer are just those which are likely to cause allergic reactions. Strawberries must come near the top of the list. If you get the occasional bout of nettle rash for no obvious reason, or even red itchy patches, which fade within a few hours, suspect a food allergy, and think back to what you've eaten in the past day.

If you are strongly allergic to any foods, you will know what they are, but slight reactions can go unrecognised. In fact, all of the berries often cause allergies. Other things which you may consume more of during the summer, and which are common allergens, are cola drinks, shellfish, pineapples, cherries and plums.

The only treatment is abstinence!

Some surprising facts you probably don't know about allergies

One teenager dies each week from asthma, 75 per cent of asthmatic children restrict their activities due to the condition.
50 per cent of asthma sufferers have disturbed sleep.
50 per cent of people with allergies lose time from work.
Allergies cause many road traffic accidents.
Exam results in Scotland and Scandinavia – where the pollen season comes later than in England – are better.
40 per cent of youngsters with allergies don't play sports.
The number of people with allergies is increasing by 5 per cent each year.

One in five people have hay fever.

Only a third of patients with allergies get any treatment.

Beware the bogus allergy tests; hair analysis, pendulums, sending spots of blood for 'radionic' tests; all are without any merit or substance. Some tests are available in health stores, from alternative practitioners, doctors interested in Clinical Ecology, and a host of so-called 'allergy experts'. None of these are scientifically proven and they are all expensive. Do not be fooled into trying them just because you're desperate. Ask yourself if they defy all common sense.

Nature's way to fight the winter ills

At the first sign of the winter frosts, we all start to take precautions – check the anti-freeze in the car and book it in for its winter service, lag the water pipes, oil the lawn mower and put it safely away for next spring, get the boiler checked and cleaned – but how many of us take the same trouble preparing our bodies for the rigours of winter?

At this time of year, how many of us get up in the morning wondering how on earth we are going to get through the day ahead? A recent survey found that 35 per cent of the population complained of winter fatigue, yet only an incredible three out of ten of them had tried to do anything about it.

Now is the time to tackle the problem. There is no need for expensive pills and potions, as in all but the worst conditions, eating the winter 'pick-me-up' foods is all you need to do.

First, take positive steps to increase your natural resistance to the bugs that thrive in central heating, on crowded buses, packed trains, and in steamy shops and offices.

Zinc and vitamin C are just two of the nutrients your body needs to keep up its defences, but even if you eat the healthy diet all the experts advise, you may be short of vital nutrients. An orange bought from the grower and freshly picked contains as much as 180 mg of vitamin C; one bought in a supermarket may not contain a single milligram.

In 1985 a survey in Britain indicated that 35 per cent of all men, and 67 per cent of all women, had an intake of zinc that fell alarmingly short of the 11 mg per day recommended by the World Health Organisation.

To ensure Super-Resistance you must know how to supplement your diet; not with pills and capsules, but with the superfoods which are extra-rich sources of the natural goodness we all need, more than ever at this time of year. After all, an ounce of prevention is worth a pound of cure.

Make sure of your vitamin A and C by eating a wide range of

foods that contain lots of both. Apples, apricots, grapes, citrus fruits, kiwi fruit, melon, pineapple and nectarines, should head your list of fruits. Try to eat at least two different ones each day.

Beetroot – with their tops – broccoli, red, green and white cabbage (raw as well as cooked), carrots, all types of cress, red, green and yellow peppers, leeks and lots of parsley, will add to your health insurance.

A good mixed diet, with some low-fat cheeses, yoghurt, meat, poultry, beans, whole grains and lots of oily fish, four eggs a week, and plenty of fresh nuts, seeds, fruits and vegetables, and you are bound to be on the right track to beat off all those winter bugs, lying in wait for the unwary.

To increase the odds in your favour, reduce the chances of winter ills and give you a genuine physical and mental boost, eat at least two of these foods each day:

Almonds These are a highly concentrated food, rich in protein and essential minerals like zinc and magnesium.

Apricots For their beta-carotene – the substance that the body converts into vitamin A – natural fruit sugar and fibre. At this time of year, good quality dried apricots are fine.

Broccoli Rich in iron, vitamins A and C, and fibre. This is not only a good winter food, but should be a regular feature on your shopping list.

Sprouted seeds The most live, pure and nutritious foods imaginable. Nothing could be fresher than harvesting your own, just before meal time. They are so easy to grow – your local health store will have the seeds and instructions – you don't even need a windowbox. They supply a powerhouse of vitamins, minerals and natural plant enzymes.

Brown rice It contains B vitamins and is a fine source of healthy calories. Serve it with stewed apples for dessert, in soups or as a substitute for potato.

Wholewheat bread A staple food for the winter months. Bursting with B vitamins and minerals, it's another provider of good calories, and hence, good energy.

Sesame seeds If there is a vegetarian in the family, then these should be a regular in your recipes. Rich in energy, protein, iron and zinc, they will give a welcome boost to all. Sprinkle them over cereals, salads, sweet or savoury dishes.

Now is the time for those wonderful home-made soups. Lots of root vegetables, onions, leeks, green veg, yeast extract and plenty of herbs and garlic. Add extra beans, lentils or barley for winter-plus nutrition.

So, don't just sit and wait for the winter ills to strike, make your shopping list right now and look forward to the spring with a new sparkle.

Now for some hints on avoiding, and dealing with, some common winter complaints.

Chilblains, those sore, itchy, inflamed and very often swollen patches of skin which mostly occur on the backs of the fingers and tops of the toes, or even on the ears, cheeks, bottom or thighs, are not only unsightly, but the pain and irritation can drive the poor unfortunate sufferer to distraction.

The principal cause of chilblains is poor circulation, and the first priority must be prevention. Caffeine, nicotine and alcohol are the three major culprits which will make your chilblains worse, as they are all vaso-constrictors – that is, substances which make blood vessels contract. Don't forget that caffeine isn't just found in tea and coffee; it's also a major component of cola drinks, including the 'diet' kind, and chocolate, whether in a cup or a box!

Smoking is just about the worst thing you can do, and if you smoke, drink lots of tea and coffee and too much booze, you are in serious trouble. Now is the time to decide if the pleasures are really worth the pain.

Extremes of temperature are another factor which can make the situation worse. Going from an overheated room or office, into sub-zero weather, causes a sudden heat loss and a consequent shutting down of the surface blood supply. The reverse is equally bad, since the rapid increase in blood flow to chilblains is what causes the maddening irritation.

Two pairs of gloves and socks will help to protect you. The inner pair should be of thinner material (silk is the best), the outer ones should be loose and thicker. Thermal socks and gloves are good, too, as are thermal long johns if you get chilblains on the thighs or legs.

Exercise is essential – yes, even in this weather. It doesn't matter what sort as long as it's regular and is brisk enough to stimulate your circulation.

Bathing with alternate hot and cold water, either in two bowls, or from a shower, or using small towels, depending on the area affected, is a great help.

If the skin of your chilblains is unbroken, add a few drops of myrrh to an eggcupful of distilled witch-hazel and rub this over the affected areas. A slice of fresh lemon dipped in sea salt can be used in the same way.

If the skin is broken, then you should use either calendula cream or comfrey ointment to soothe the pain and to encourage faster healing. Aloe vera gel is another good alternative.

To help with the circulation, 400 units of vitamin E and 1 g of vitamin C with bioflavinoids should be taken each day, together with a good vitamin B complex.

The commonest cause of winter muscle pain is fibrositis, an inflammation of muscle fibres. Small nodules of fibrous tissue arise deep in the large muscles, and, like the sand in an oyster, irritate surrounding muscle fibres so that they, too, knot up. The fibrous nodules grow larger and larger and eventually produce severe pain and discomfort. Fibrositis usually occurs in the large muscles of the neck, shoulders, back and buttocks, but can occur in any muscle subject to undue stress and strain.

Any osteopath or masseur – practitioners who have their hands on patients all the time – can pinpoint the areas of muscle responsible for pain purely through their well-developed sense of touch.

Whatever the type of muscle or joint pain, two things which you can always do to help yourself are to keep your weight down and to keep as active as is appropriate for your age and physical condition. Adding a cup of Epsom salts or Radox herbal extract to a hot bath, and soaking in it for a quarter of an hour, will help. So, too, will gentle and alternating hot and cold compresses. A herbal anti-inflammatory like Bio-Strath willow formula reduces the pain and has no side effects, so is worth a try.

It may seem surprising, but changing your diet can bring about marked improvements. Cut out all red meat and meat products. Eat lots of oily fish like herrings, sardines, mackerel, pilchards, salmon and tuna. Eat more green vegetables, less sugar and drink much less tea and coffee. Cut out all the citrus fruits (oranges, lemons and grapefruit). These changes reduce the 'acidity' of the system, and though most scientists argue with this concept, Naturopaths have applied these ideas for many years and with good results.

A daily dose of 2000 mg of calcium pantothenate should be taken when the pain is acute. Once you start to feel better it should be reduced to 500 mg, then lowered gradually to 50 mg daily. Zinc, calcium and magnesium are essential for good muscle function, so a tablet of Magnesium-OK should also be taken each day.

Winter is that time of year when the flu virus is most likely to be on the rampage, and there is no point in saying 'I never get it.' Each year there are changes in the virus, and at some point you will come into contact with a particular strain that your defence system has not met before. You will have little or no resistance to it, and you will succumb.

This does not mean that you just sit back and wait to be struck down, far from it. Start now, to improve the strength of your immune system, which will provide greater protection and will help to make your dose of the dreaded flu as mild as possible. With luck and a little healthy living, you may avoid flu altogether.

Have you ever stopped to wonder why it is that some people seem to resist all the infections that come and go, whilst others seem to catch them all? Why does the person at the next desk in the office escape each bout of flu, and every stomach bug, when no one else does?

Good nutrition is the key to a sound immune system, so you must try to maintain a balanced, mixed diet in order to ensure an adequate intake of all the essential vitamins, minerals and trace elements. Day and night, the body has to combat all kinds of disease-causing organisms, and if your body has an adequate defence mechanism, then when the winter flu bugs are spreading like wildfire, your chances of going under will be greatly reduced.

You need plenty of citrus fruits for their vitamin C, lots of seeds and nuts for vitamin E and minerals, particularly pumpkin seeds for their high content of zinc: as much fresh salad, vegetables and all other fruit as you can eat, together with good cereals and protein, from fish and poultry.

As an extra insurance policy, it is a good idea to take Bio-Strath Elixir – this has been proved to increase the number of the vital 'T-helper cells' in the blood, and a simple multivitamin like Genesis, each day during the winter months.

If you are unlucky enough to fall foul of the flu bug, then here is a quick-action plan to get you back on your feet in record time.

First Day

On rising: A glass of Evian water.

Breakfast: One teaspoonful of Bio-Strath, juice of half a grapefruit in half a glass of hot water, topped up with apple juice, and a dessertspoon of honey, a bunch of grapes; an apple, and a sprinkle of cinnamon.

Mid-morning: A glass of hot water and honey, with a sprinkle of cinnamon; a few grapes.

Lunch: One teaspoonful of Bio-Strath, a large glass of Evian water; a large bowl of dried fruit – apricots, figs, sultanas, etc. – which you covered with boiling water the previous evening, and left to soak overnight; squeeze a little lemon juice into it, and add a teaspoon of sesame seeds and a dessertspoon of pumpkin seeds.

Mid-afternoon: Another drink; hot blackcurrant and apple juice (natural, not sweetened) with a little honey and half a teaspoon of dried ginger.

Evening: One teaspoonful of Bio-Strath, a mixed salad of fresh raw vegetables – cabbage finely shredded, lettuce, grated carrot, celeriac, cucumber, grated raw beetroot, fennel, watercress, whatever is fresh and in season – with a dressing of virgin olive oil, lemon juice, two crushed cloves of fresh garlic, chopped onions and parsley. Fresh fruit – especially mango, papaya, or pineapple – and a large glass of Evian water.

Bed time: A large glass of hot water, with a teaspoon of honey, ginger and a slice of lemon.

Second Day

On rising: Same as First Day until evening.

Evening: One teaspoonful of Bio-Strath. A mixed salad with the dressing as above *plus* a medium baked potato and some sugar-free baked beans.

Bed time: Hot water as before.

Third Day

On rising: A large glass of Evian water.

Breakfast: One teaspoonful of Bio-Strath. Start preparing this the night before. Put a couple of spoonfuls of oatflakes in a cereal bowl, add a tablespoonful of water and leave to soak overnight. In the morning, stir in a teaspoonful of fresh lemon juice, a carton of low-fat, live yoghurt and a small banana. A cup of weak tea, preferably China or chamomile.

Mid-morning: A big glass of vegetable juice – freshly pressed if possible – or canned or bottled juices which are salt-free.

Then back to the 'flu-fighter' Better Eating Plan as above. Don't make the mistake of going back to work too soon – flu is a serious problem and can leave you weak, depressed and more vulnerable to subsequent infections. So take extra care of yourself, and let nature's store-house help build better resistance.

A sore throat can strike at any time. It is Murphy's Law that when you get one, it couldn't come at a worse time.

The first step in the relief of any sore throat is to drink large amounts of liquid. Water, diluted pineapple juice or cool chamomile tea, are the best. A cold, damp compress, wrapped around the neck, is very soothing. This is just as good for small children as it is for adults, so don't be tempted to use hot towels, or water bottles, no matter how appealing they may seem.

I always ask my patients with throat problems to change their eating habits for a day or so. This may sound strange, but it works. For the first twenty-four hours eat only fresh fruit, and drink nothing but fresh fruit juice or water. (This is not suitable for children under two.) Follow this with a few days of mainly fruit, vegetables, salads and light protein like fish or poultry. Avoid dairy products, as they encourage the body to produce more mucus, and use only small amounts of starch, and *no* sugar, until the symptoms have gone.

If your throat is part of a rotten cold, stay in the warm, keep the air moist by using a humidifier or a bowl of water on top of the radiator. Inhale the vapours of 'Climarome', a herbal, aroma-therapy product, made by the leading French expert, Dr Valnet – available from good health stores or chemists. Spray it on your pillow and handkerchief, as well as into the air in your bedroom. Friar's Balsam is good too, if you are chesty.

Gargles are an essential part of the treatment. Here are two of the ones which I prescribe most often:

Make an infusion of sage and thyme, using half a teaspoon of each dried herb, or one teaspoon of fresh, chopped leaves of each. Pour half a pint of boiling water on the herbs, cover, and leave to stand for ten minutes. Then pour the infusion through a tea-strainer, wait till it is cool enough to use comfortably, then gargle thoroughly with the whole quantity. Repeat this four or five times a day, but do not swallow the gargle. If you are not making revolting and disgusting noises at the back of your throat, then you aren't doing it right!

Hot water, honey and lemon juice make another favourite gargle. Two tablespoonsful of honey, the juice of a large lemon, and half a pint of hot water. Use it as above, but this time swallow the mixture. It is too good to waste.

A good drink for sore throats can be made by warming a little red wine, to which you add a tablespoon of honey, a pinch of cinnamon, two cloves, one clove of garlic and a thick slice of lemon. It is great as a bedtime drink, though it is a little anti-social.

Take plenty of vitamin C, at least 1 g daily, and suck four zinc and vitamin C tablets a day, as these will act directly on the painful membranes.

Persistent sore throats should not be ignored, and any sudden changes in the voice, which don't get better after a few days, should be investigated by your GP. But using these simple self-help remedies will avoid lots of antibiotics, which you don't often need for the treatment of a simple sore throat.

As soon as winter comes and the temperature starts to drop, the papers are full of stories about hypothermia. We are all told to look out for elderly neighbours, watch for milk left on the doorstep, papers still in the letterbox, drawn curtains in the middle of the day, and the other tell-tale signs that all is not well. And so we should, without reminders from the media, and throughout the year, not just in winter.

Why is it that more old people die of heart attacks in the winter here in the UK than in countries that have far more severe weather than we do? The medical reason is that when the body temperature drops, the blood gets thicker. The heart must work harder to pump it round the body, and this extra effort is sometimes enough to overload an already weakened heart.

The social reasons are much more interesting, easier to do something about, and they apply to all of us, regardless of age.

In the really cold countries like Scandinavia, Switzerland, and parts of Eastern Europe, they do not have the British 'stiff upper lip' attitude to the cold. They accept that there is such a thing as weather, and behave accordingly. We Brits spend a great deal of energy talking about it, but at the same time pretend that it does not exist. We leave our centrally heated houses, and stand at the bus stop for half an hour in sub-zero temperatures, while the howling wind chills us even more. Do we wear a thick woolly hat – fur-lined gloves and boots – thermal undies – ear-muffs – long scarves – lots of layers of clothes? No, we don't. We tend to put on an extra sweater, possibly a thin pair of gloves, a coat and an umbrella to keep off the snow.

The cure is so simple, anyone can do it. You can be one of the walking warm this winter. There is weather, so gear up for it. Ignore the fashion pundits, dress for comfort and health. Keep head, hands and feet warm, and stride out, facing the elements full frontal. Stand tall, chest out, stomach in, head high, and walk. Do not slouch, amble or creep.

The secret is to get your circulation, and your breathing, working hard. Muscular activity generates heat – your sensible winter clothes will keep it next to your body, where it's needed – and walking warm will get your blood flowing, and your lungs working overtime.

Double glazing, better insulation and central heating tend to isolate us from the elements; even more so if home is several floors up in a block of flats. By the time you get outside, and realise how cold it is, you can't be bothered to go back to get some warm clothes. I advise my patients to buy a thermometer, and fix it outside the kitchen window. Get into the habit of looking at it before you get dressed to go out in the winter.

Finally, you might not expect me to advocate alcoholic drinks, but a small tipple is no bad thing in the depths of winter. A glass of hot mulled wine is just the ticket. Heat the red wine, put a sachet of

255

'Country House' spice mixture into your glass, add the wine and
enjoy the warming benefits of cinnamon, cloves, aniseed, fennel
and the circulatory stimulus of the wine. After all, that's what
they do on top of the Swiss mountains. At this time of the year,
your skin has to contend with all those winter hazards; some you
can avoid, others you'll have to learn how to live with and
compensate for.

Good food is vital at all times of the year, but even more so during
the winter months. Icy winds that blast away the natural oils from
your skin; central heating that dries out the essential moisture;
sudden changes from the hot office or home, to the freezing great
outdoors, which may damage the delicate and tiny blood vessels just
below the surface; jobs that have to be done outside and in all
weathers, and chap and chafe your hands and face; lack of sunlight,
which means less vitamin D – these are the external factors with
which your skin has to contend.

The internal factors are connected to your diet – less fresh fruit,
salads and vegetables (much of what we eat at this time of year has
been stored for some time and this depletes its vitamin content).

All this spells disaster for your skin: red blotchy patches, dry,
scaly and flaking areas that spread over the cheeks and forehead;
red veins around the nose and cheek bones, dry and split lips, with
cracks at the corners of the mouth; ugly and swollen cracks and
chaps on the hands and flaky, ridged and split finger nails.

If all this sounds familiar, then here's your action plan for
beautiful winter skin.

Make sure that you eat lots of these special skin foods, packed
with the nutrients your skin needs for extra winter protection:

Carrots for their high vitamin A content, the most important of
all the vitamins for skin; avocado pears which protect the skin by
their antioxidant vitamins A and E, and also help the body produce
more collagen to keep the skin supple; oats for their vitamins B and
E, and lots of vital minerals; sprouted seeds, a must during the
winter, for they are packed full of super skin nutrients and are
always fresh when you want them.

So much for the inside, but how about some external protection?
Next to fresh air and sunlight, keeping your skin clean is the most
important thing you can do. If you have a sensitive skin, then it is
best to avoid the strongly perfumed soaps and rather stick to natural
non-animal ones.

Avoid the medicated soaps which may kill off the good bugs as
well as the bad. Never add antiseptics or disinfectants to the bath,
and don't use bubble bath or crystals, as these tend to dry out the
skin. At this time of year it needs all the moisture it can get.
Oatmeal soap, natural bath oils and lots of moisturiser are the first
steps to glowing winter skin. Use a daily application of aloe vera gel

to the hands and face, and calendula (marigold) cream to soothe cracked or itchy areas.

Hands are very vulnerable, so make sure that you wear gloves for washing up, housework, gardening and whenever you go out in the cold. One capsule of evening primrose oil can be pierced, then squeezed onto the hands and massaged into the skin at bedtime.

To give that extra bad weather insurance, take 7500 units of vitamin A and 1 g of evening primrose oil, daily during the winter months.

For hands that are as soft as your face, follow these tips and protect your skin from the ravages of the weather this winter.

How to survive Christmas

With the best will in the world, we all tend to indulge in too much merry making during the Christmas holiday. And, after every Lord Mayor's Show, comes the day of reckoning: stomachs bulging with a surfeit of food, livers awash with alcohol, eyes bleary after hours in front of the telly, all-in-all, a sad and sorry state.

It's no good crying over spilt port and mince pies. You've got to do something so that you can face the future with more than a sore head. I know that you are dreaming about those New Year's resolutions, but dreaming won't help now. What you need is an immediate action plan, and here it is.

Mince pies, plum-pudding, sage and onion stuffing, mulled wine and ale, Christmas cake, ginger wine, apple and spice and all things nice: they all add up to the Christmas binge.

But take heart, or rather stomach. All is not lost. Of course it makes sense to try to be just a bit restrained during this festive season, but you can't say no each time you get offered a drink or a mince pie. Salvation is at hand in the shape of all the herbs and spices that we use at this time of the year.

When our forefathers quaffed their Yuletide tankards of spicy wine and beer they were indeed drinking to their own 'good health'.

All those warming tropical spices that crop up in our traditional Christmas foods – cinnamon, nutmeg, cloves, ginger – help us to digest the extra-rich fare and they are a great herbal shot in the arm for cold weather vitality.

Cloves A good aid to digestion. They help to stimulate the circulation, and increase resistance to infection. So they keep at bay the winter chill and chills.

Cinnamon Will warm the whole body. It relieves indigestion and even combats the toxic after-effects of overindulgence. If the stomach or bowels are in trouble, then you need cinnamon.

257

If you are unlucky enough to feel a cold coming on right at the start of the holiday, try this soothing prescription: Stir a quarter of a teaspoon of ground cinnamon into a glass of hot water, add the juice of a lemon and a dessertspoon of honey. Sip slowly at bedtime.

Nutmeg   Should be a constant companion at this time of the year. It is a staunch ally of your digestive system, which is why traditional recipes for rich cakes and puddings include it.

Ginger   Does just what you would expect; it 'gingers up' your whole system. The digestion and circulation are most affected by this amazing spice. And if you are sluggish, bloated and post-festive, try a good pinch of powdered ginger or some freshly grated root ginger in a small glass of hot water. This mixture should be sipped slowly.

Once Christmas is out of the way, the trials and tribulations of the New Year are instantly upon you. Revitalise your poor overworked system with this Body Talk 24-hour 'body treat'.

Start your day with a large glass of hot water containing the juice of a lemon. For breakfast, some exotic fruits – fresh pineapple, mango, pawpaw, kiwi and passion fruit. Drink a cup or two of mint tea, then off for a brisk half-hour walk. The vitamin C and enzymes in the fruit will start the process of repair and cleansing that your body needs.

Mid-morning, have another glass of water and lemon, with a snack of raisins, dates, sultanas and a handful of fresh nuts, which replace essential minerals, and give you a lift from the natural sugar in the dried fruits.

Lunch should be a large mixed salad. Make sure you include plenty of raw carrot, cabbage, red and yellow peppers, and watercress, together with the normal ingredients. This ensures a high intake of vitamin A and iron. Sprinkle a heaped teaspoon of sesame seeds over the top (they are rich in zinc, which your depleted defences need), and serve with a dressing of extra virgin olive oil, with a dash of lemon juice, two crushed cloves of garlic and a teaspoon of honey. Drink at least two glasses of plain water.

The natural bacteria, which live in your intestines, do not take too kindly to alcohol, so replace them by an afternoon nibble of a pot of natural yoghurt, mixed with a tablespoon of honey, and treat yourself to a cup of weak tea.

The evening meal is high in fibre, vitamins and minerals. It is designed to provide plenty of bulk, so you won't feel hungry, but is easy to digest. Have a selection of lightly cooked vegetables. Do include some root vegetables as well, they are rich in minerals. Eat these with a large jacket potato, served with some natural yoghurt and chives. Drink plenty of water and keep away from all those boxes of chocolates! You'll feel like a new person in the morning.

The traditional Christmas cold is nearly as traditional as the holly. Often a result of the long period of overeating, drinking and high living. The body uses the cold as a way of getting rid of some of the extra junk that has been stuffed into it. You should try to encourage this natural method of elimination and not suppress it.

There is a mixture which Victorian herbalists swore by. It will open the pores, raise the temperature and free the mucus!

To make this magic elixir all you need is a quarter of a teaspoon of cayenne pepper, stir it into a small glass of hot water, sweeten with a teaspoon of honey and down it in one gulp. The feeling is just a bit worse than 100 proof vodka, but the good it'll do you is worth it. If you take this cure during the day, make sure that you wrap up well before you go out into the cold winter air.

At night put an extra blanket on the bed and tuck yourself in with a hot water bottle. Prepare for a hot and sweaty night as the cayenne starts to work the cold out of your system.

If you want a hearty and healthy way to see in the New Year, here's my favourite spice punch. Put the juice of a large orange into a stainless steel, enamel or glass pan. Add the thinly sliced peel of the orange, a cupful of water, a tablespoon of honey and another large orange, well washed and stuck with a dozen cloves.

Now put in a whole cinnamon stick, a generous grating of nutmeg, bring to the boil and simmer for twenty minutes. Add a bottle of red wine – not cheap plonk, but not your best vintage either – and serve piping hot. For the children's party you can use a couple of cartons of apple, pear or grape juice. The parents will enjoy it as much as the kids.

Finally, watch out for the 'telly belly' – that grumbling, rumbling discomfort which seems to infect the whole family after the large meals on Christmas Day and Boxing Day. You stagger from the table, fall into your favourite chair and are instantly mesmerised by the TV screen.

Don't do it. Give your poor, overworked stomach a sporting chance by taking it for a stroll round the block or into the park. That at least will give your digestion some time to get to work on its vast overload before you settle down to the mince pies, nuts and raisins.

Gold, Frankincense and Myrrh may have been the original gifts, but Cinnamon, Cloves and Ginger will spice up your life at Christmas.

A three-week slimming plan

First Week

Monday
    Breakfast: Half grapefruit, raw apple, China tea and lemon
    Lunch: Cream of celery soup, mixed salad, 2 Ryvita, grapes
    Dinner: Steamed carrots, Brussels sprouts, cheese sauce, baked
        apple

Tuesday
    Breakfast: Grapes, orange, China tea and lemon
    Lunch: Tomato soup, large salad, 2 Ryvita, prunes
    Dinner: Baked potato, little butter on potato, small mixed salad,
        pear

Wednesday
    Breakfast: Stewed apple, pear, China tea and lemon
    Lunch: Large mixed salad, baked potato, butter, fresh fruit
    Dinner: Vegetable soup, French beans, carrots, parsnips, butter
        sauce, baked apple

Thursday
    Breakfast: Baked apple, half grapefruit, China tea and lemon
    Lunch: Large mixed salad, 2 Ryvita, butter, stewed pears
    Dinner: Tomato juice, carrots, cheese sauce, baked apple

Friday
    Breakfast: Prunes, grapes, China tea and lemon
    Lunch: Cream of celery soup, large mixed salad, 2 Ryvita, butter,
        raw apple
    Dinner: Apple juice, baked potato, butter beans, spinach,
        stewed apple

Saturday
    Breakfast: Half grapefruit, raw apple, China tea and lemon
    Lunch: Vegetable soup, mixed salad, 2 Ryvita, butter, pear
    Dinner: Tomato juice, carrots, beans, small salad, fruit salad

Sunday
    Breakfast: Stewed apple, pear, China tea and lemon

Lunch: Large mixed salad, baked potato, butter, fresh fruit
Dinner: Vegetable soup, French beans, carrots, parsnips, butter
      sauce, fruit salad

Note
(1) Mid-morning, mid-afternoon and during the evening a cup of
    VECON (obtainable from health food stores), China tea or
    very weak Indian tea should be taken and at least three large
    glasses of water.
(2) A large mixed salad consists of lettuce, tomatoes, grated raw
    carrots, grated cooked beetroot, celery, raw onion, chopped
    apple, watercress and any other raw vegetables or salad
    produce you like.
(3) A dressing of lemon or cider vinegar and sunflower or safflower
    oil can be used on the salad.
(4) Add a dessertspoon of bran to the soup or yoghurt.

Second Week
Monday
    Breakfast: Orange, prunes, yoghurt
    Lunch: Tomato juice, large mixed salad, baked potato, butter,
       grapes
    Dinner: Celery soup, carrots, sprouts, beans, cheese sauce, fruit
       salad

Tuesday
    Breakfast: Half grapefruit, apple, yoghurt
    Lunch: Apple juice, large mixed salad, 2 Ryvita, butter, baked
       apple
    Dinner: Tomato juice, spinach, baked parsnips, carrots, butter
       sauce, pear

Wednesday
    Breakfast: Grapes, apple, yoghurt
    Lunch: Tomato soup, large mixed salad, baked potato, stewed
       pears
    Dinner: Half grapefruit, celery, cauliflower, beans, cheese sauce,
       some kind of fruit

Thursday
    Breakfast: Pear, baked apple, yoghurt
    Lunch: Apple juice, large mixed salad, 2 Ryvita, prunes
    Dinner: Tomato juice, baked potato, sprouts, carrots, butter
       sauce, grapes

Friday
    Breakfast: Orange, pear, yoghurt

Lunch: Celery soup, large mixed salad, Ryvita, butter, stewed raisins.
Dinner: Tomato juice, celery, cauliflower, baked parsnips, cheese sauce, raw apple

Saturday
Breakfast: Half grapefruit, apple, yoghurt
Lunch: Apple juice, large mixed salad, baked potato, butter, stewed apple
Dinner: Vegetable soup, beans, celery, sprouts, cheese sauce, fruit salad

Sunday
Breakfast: Grapes, apple, yoghurt
Lunch: Tomato soup, large mixed salad, baked potato, stewed pears
Dinner: Half grapefruit, celery, cauliflower, beans, cheese sauce, some kind of fresh fruit

---

Third Week
Continue as the Second Week with the addition to the dinners of fish twice a week, chicken twice a week. For the remaining three days, the evening meal should stay vegetarian. Any vegetarian protein may be used instead of fish or chicken.

Dieting can be bad for your sleep

Without doubt, one of the most commonly held beliefs about fat and thin people is that the first are happy and the second less so. This conception is enshrined in our literary heritage. You only need to compare the ebullient, jolly, roly-poly Mr Pickwick with the lean and hungry Cassius. Both Dickens and Shakespeare understood this difference and exploited it widely. Just consider Scrooge and Falstaff, Uriah Heep and Mistress Quickly. Writers and playwrights and even – in more modern times – the creators of television series have drawn on this fundamental difference in order to highlight two extremes of the human condition.

Despite the efforts of the slimming lobby to persuade us that all overweight people are, in truth, desperately miserable and unhappy thinnies struggling to get out of their fat shells, and the tireless attempts of the advertising industry to project all that is good, beautiful, desirable and aspirational as thin, Shakespeare and Dickens got it just about right.

We have seen already that anxious people sleep less well than happy ones (see Insomnia). We also know that happy people have better appetites and a better ability to absorb food than those suffering from anxiety. The happy bunch inevitably have a tendency to gain weight, whilst the unhappy are more likely to lose it, sometimes even unwittingly.

As always, there are exceptions that prove the rule, and occasionally the response to anxiety, stress and unhappiness is 'comfort eating' and subsequent weight gain. This, though, is far less common.

The scientific link between weight and sleep was first described in a paper published in the British Medical Journal in 1976 by Professor Arthur Crisp. He and his researchers conducted a random survey of 1000 men and women. They were all weighed and asked a selection of questions with the object of determining how they felt about themselves, specifically in relation to anxiety and depression. The end result showed that the overweight members of the group were more satisfied with life and generally of a happier disposition than their thinner counterparts. Happiness is equated with sleeping well, whereas anxiety and depression almost inevitably lead to sleep of less quality and more disruption.

Overall, the overweight slept for longer and they enjoyed proportionately more paradoxical sleep. It is during this phase of sleep that the greatest degree of muscular relaxation occurs – waking from paradoxical sleep frequently results in momentary sensations of paralysis – and more paradoxical sleep means renewed energy the following day.

There is no denying that the thin, over-anxious, tense person is far more likely to suffer from sleep problems. Overcoming the root cause of the anxiety and depression is a prerequisite to improving sleep habits. These mental anxiety states are frequently the result of an inability to cope with the demands of life but appropriate psychotherapy will usually resolve the problems in time.

Faulty eating habits, on the other hand, can produce far more intractable problems and this is even more so in self-inflicted nutritional deprivation. There is currently a vogue for a whole range of extreme dietary regimes, none of them healthy, none of them with any basis in sound scientific fact and none of them to be recommended. Whether an individual takes it upon himself to follow some absurd guru, or whether dietary changes are recommended directly by any one of the myriad of alternative health practitioners, the end result will be the same.

It is rare to see obvious clinical signs of malnutrition in this country, save in the case of anorexia nervosa, but more of that later. What is disturbingly common is the incidence of 'sub-clinical' malnutrition – that is, the accumulated deficit in essential nutrients which is not enough to cause scurvy, rickets or beri-beri, but is sufficient to interfere with the efficient workings of the body's biological machine. This disturbance of function almost invariably leads to disturbance of sleep.

Why do people embark on these ridiculous diets? Sometimes out of pure vanity, sometimes through social pressures imposed by peers, occupational demands or even family interference. They may have been told they suffer from food allergies; they may have been prescribed an outrageous diet for the treatment of candida (a condition which, though currently fashionable in alternative medicine circles, has yet to be supported by a shred of medical evidence in the majority of cases).

Beware the so-called nutritionists who are not complementary practitioners, nor alternative practitioners. They're not even fringe practitioners; they are beyond the fringe. Most of them boast worthless diplomas graciously bestowed in return for large amounts of money by establishments whose prime objective is to train salesmen and women in the art of foisting their own particular products onto an unsuspecting public in the guise of nutritional counselling. These people play on the emotions of an unsuspecting public. One recently reported case was that of a teenage boy who developed epilepsy. The parents, not wishing to accept this diagnosis, grasped at the straw of beyond the fringe medicine, a practitioner of which diagnosed their son as having food allergies. He was put on a very restricted diet which produced no improvement. They took him to another practitioner, who removed even more foods from his diet. By the time he'd been to the third charlatan he was living exclusively on five different foods.

When admitted to hospital he was suffering from severe scurvy and hours from death. And, of course, he still had his epilepsy. This is an extreme story, but a warning to those who decide to follow ridiculous dietary regimes based on bogus diagnoses and prescribed by totally unqualified and irresponsible practitioners. Just because you are faced with a man in a white coat with a row of glossy diplomas (mostly not worth the paper they're printed on), don't suspend your own powers of critical judgement or common sense.

Anorexia nervosa is a completely different situation and one which needs intensive psychiatric intervention and psychological counselling. As in all situations of nutritional deprivation, sleep patterns are affected early on. It is well documented that as dieters lose weight, they sleep less. This pattern is not so much a reflection of the quantity of food being eaten, but of the total body weight.

Studies on anorexics show that at the beginning of treatment, although they were being fed a good diet but were still very thin, they tended to fall asleep normally but wake up very early and were unable to get back to sleep. As their weight increased, the length of time they stayed asleep gradually increased and by the time their weight was normal, so was their sleep.

The moral is clear: if you are already suffering from insomnia, don't go on a weight-loss diet. If you are underweight, putting on a few pounds will help to improve your sleep. If you are overweight with a sleep problem, this is not the time to think about reducing, unless of course there are serious medical reasons why you should – heart disease, severe breathing problems or if you're awaiting surgery.

Severe obesity, on the other hand, can also interfere with your sleep. It adversely affects breathing, increases the likelihood of disruptive snoring and may lead to sleep apnoea. Carrying excessive weight encourages degenerative arthritic changes in the weight-bearing joints, spine, hips, knees and ankles. Arthritis is extremely painful, and pain disrupts sleep. If you do need to lose weight, make sure you follow a sensible dietary regime. Do not use very low-calorie meal replacements, mono-diets or any extreme eating plan which does not supply you with a full spectrum of food sources or sufficient calories to enable you to carry on with your normal daily activities.

Never go to bed hungry, and never go to bed on an overfull stomach. Too little food and that gnawing pang in the pit of your stomach will certainly make sure that you have a restless night of fitful sleep. Too much and you will suffer indigestion, heartburn, flatulence and again a disturbed night. If you suffer from an hiatus hernia you need to take special care with your evening eating habits. This condition, in which the opening in the diaphragm through which the oesophagus (food tube) passes becomes too loose and allows the acid contents of the stomach to leak upwards into the oesophagus, causes most disruption at night time. As soon as you lie down, the presence of stomach acids in the wrong place causes severe heartburn and considerable pain. There are practical steps which minimise this disruptive discomfort. Raise the head end of your bed by about 4 inches using proper bed blocks or a brick under each leg. Do not drink any liquids at all less than three hours before bedtime. Do not eat large meals in the evening. And avoid pickles, vinegar, acidic foods and anything fried.

There is some evidence that malted milk drinks like Horlicks and Ovaltine really do help to encourage better sleep. The beneficial effects are more apparent in older people, and the main benefits seem to be during the later stages of sleep rather than in getting to sleep in the first place. If you find that you drop off easily, but wake in the small hours, it's certainly worth trying either of these drinks about half an hour before bedtime.

Honey has long been a favourite folk remedy for insomnia. Take it mixed with a little warm milk, in a cup of chamomile tea or in hot water with lemon. And don't forget all the other soothing herbal remedies.

There is no denying that we are what we eat and you cannot expect a good night's sleep if you are constantly consuming large quantities of coffee, tea, chocolate or cola drinks, which all supply your brain with a constant stream of irritating caffeine. You won't sleep if you're hungry. You're unlikely to sleep after a take-away snack of pie, chips and three pickled onions. As far as food is concerned, the watch-words should be: not too little, not too much, but just right. What is just right for you, you will find by trial and error.

Food intolerance or food allergy?
A vexed question

Over the last few years enormous media coverage has been given to the subject of food allergies. You've all read about people suffering from total allergy syndrome: being allergic not only to food, water and many of the additives used in food processing, but to the world we live in – petrol fumes, polluted air, tap water. I have even seen patients who have been told by so-called allergy experts that they are allergic to themselves. The mushrooming boom in allergy clinics and the growing number of allergy testing techniques which vary from pendulum swinging to absent diagnosis, to say nothing of the pseudo-scientific mumbo-jumbo which daily gains in popularity, have all served to make a large number of people totally obsessed with what they eat, drink, breathe, wear, or even where they live.

Whilst there are very specific allergic reactions to some foods, particularly shellfish, eggs, milk and even some fruits like strawberries, the vast majority of people who develop side effects from eating foods do not suffer from allergies. These people present what are much better called adverse food reactions, or food intolerance.

Some half of the world's population do not produce the enzyme necessary to digest milk, therefore it is not surprising that many people can show evidence of milk intolerance, especially that produced by lactose intolerance. (Lactose is the name of the sugar which occurs naturally in milk.) Apart from milk, other foods which can produce adverse effects in a wide range of people include coffee, tea, cocoa, chocolate, cheese, beer, sausages, some canned foods, yeast, red wine, wheat, and even tomatoes.

Specific individuals may have an intolerance to many other food substances, and the list of illnesses which can be aggravated or even caused by these food intolerances is wide ranging. Migraine, asthma, eczema, urticaria, irritable bowel syndrome, colitis, Crohn's disease, hay fever, rheumatoid arthritis, are just some conditions which may respond to quite drastic changes in diet. Add to this list premenstrual syndrome and menopausal problems and you have a range of illnesses which affect a vast proportion of people at some time or other during their lives.

Some of these conditions will respond to the exclusion of certain foods from the diet. For example, skin conditions like eczema and urticaria usually respond well to diets which exclude all milk and dairy products, eggs and the foods which naturally contain salicylates together with those used in food preserving, colouring and flavouring, especially tartrazine. The other conditions are often caused by a much wider range of food intolerances and for that reason it is best to start with an exclusion diet.

The exclusion diet

Although at first sight this diet looks horrendously difficult for anyone to follow, do remember that you only need to follow it rigorously for about two weeks, after which foods may be added to the diet and, provided you keep an accurate record of what you add, when you add it and what the results are, you will soon be able to build up a relatively wide spectrum of foods to which you are tolerant and eliminate those to which you are intolerant.

Dr John Hunter and Dr Virginia Alun Jones, together with dietician Elizabeth Workman, working at Addenbrooke's Hospital in Cambridge, have produced an excellent book on these problems called *The Allergy Diet* and the following scheme is based on their hospital research in Cambridge.

Do keep an exact record of everything you eat and drink, together with any symptoms which you may notice, for one week before you start the diet. During the first two weeks of the diet you must stick to it exactly as outlined and even one day's lapse will undo all the work you have done so far, and you will need to start again.

In addition to excluding all the foods listed, you should also exclude any foods which you know or even suspect may upset you personally. It is important to eat as wide a variety of the permitted foods as you can, since even those on the permitted list can cause adverse reactions in some people and it will help if you discover these early on. Throughout this fortnight do keep your diary again, so that you can discover if any of the foods you are eating are affecting you adversely.

After two weeks, you should notice dramatic improvements in your health. If your symptoms have not improved, then food intolerance is probably not the cause of your problems and you should seek further nutritional guidance from a naturopath.

The following are the foods which you may and may not eat during the first two weeks of the exclusion diet:

	Not allowed	Allowed
Meat	preserved meats, bacon, sausages	all other meats

Fish	smoked fish, shellfish	white fish
Vegetables	potatoes, onions, sweetcorn	all other vegetables, salads, pulses, swede and parsnip
Fruit	citrus fruit, e.g. oranges, grapefruit	all other fruit, e.g. apples, bananas, pears
Cereals	wheat, oats, barley, rye, corn	rice, ground rice, rice flakes, rice flour, sago, Rice Krispies, tapioca, millet, buckwheat, rice cakes
Cooking oils	corn oil, vegetable oil	sunflower oil, soya oil, safflower oil, olive oil
Dairy products	cow's milk, butter, most margarines, yoghurt and cheese, eggs	goat's milk, soya milk, sheep's milk, Tomor margarine, goat's and sheep's milk yoghurt and cheese, soya cheese
Beverages	tea, coffee (beans, instant and decaffeinated), fruit squashes, orange juice, grapefruit juice, alcohol, tap water	herbal teas (e.g. chamomile), fresh fruit juices (e.g. apple, pineapple), tomato juice, mineral, distilled or de-ionised water
Miscellaneous	chocolates, yeast, preservatives	carob, sea salt, herbs, spices; in moderation: sugar, honey

You should make sure that you buy fresh or freshly frozen foods, since tinned and packeted foods are likely to contain the additives to which you may well be sensitive. Also beware of many prepared foods, especially biscuits, cakes, cake mixes, puddings, and most sweets and chocolates, since these are likely to contain milk or milk products.

At the end of the fortnight you can start to reintroduce some other food varieties. Continue to keep your diet diary so that you can record any mishaps and introduce foods in the order listed below and advocated by Drs Hunter and Jones in their book:

(1) Tap water
(2) Potatoes
(3) Cow's milk
(4) Yeast

(5) Tea
(6) Rye
(7) Butter
(8) Onions
(9) Eggs
(10) Porridge oats
(11) Coffee
(12) Chocolate
(13) Barley
(14) Citrus fruits
(15) Corn
(16) Cow's cheese
(17) White wine
(18) Shellfish
(19) Natural cow's milk yoghurt
(20) Vinegar
(21) Wheat
(22) Nuts
(23) Preservatives (this is one which I personally would recommend my patients to avoid in any case as far as possible)

Do not introduce any one new food item in any two-day period. If you have any obvious reaction, stop eating that particular food, make a note and carry on to the next food once all reactions have settled down. Do drink plenty of water and try to avoid taking any form of medication unless this is specifically prescribed by your doctor and essential.

Many people have created more problems than they have solved by careless use of exclusion diets, either through trying to do it themselves or through ill-informed and bad advice from supposed allergy practitioners. Unless you eat a wide spread of nutrients it is quite possible to end up suffering not only from the symptoms which you are trying to alleviate, but also from malnutrition. The above is a guide to exclusion diets and not a complete and detailed set of instructions. For these you need to read the full text of *The Allergy Diet* and you will need the help and guidance of a competent naturopath or dietician.

The Hay diet

Dr William Howard Hay was one of the great pioneers of the food reform movement. After suffering severe ill health himself and getting no relief from his doctors in America at the turn of the century, he decided to take matters into his own hands and to treat his condition by making radical changes to his diet. He decided to eat only such things as he believed were intended by nature as food for man, taking them in natural form and in quantities no greater than seemed necessary for his present need. This return to fundamental eating produced dramatic changes in his health and after three months he had returned to his former vigour. He then applied the same principles to treating his own patients and finally in his book *A New Health Era* outlined the principles of the Hay system of eating.

Before the First World War Hay suggested that the over-consumption of white flour products, refined sugar and other refined carbohydrates, the eating of too much meat and constipation were vital factors in the cause of many digestive disorders and other health complaints. How interesting that the most up-to-date thinking on nutrition and health implicates the same factors as well as others. In their book *Food Combining For Health* Doris Grant and Jean Joyce take a new look at the Hay system and provide a detailed and fascinating account of the remarkably beneficial effects of changing to this pattern of eating.

They have extracted Hay's five important principles: (1) starches and sugars should not be eaten with proteins and acid fruits at the same meal; (2) vegetables, salads and fruits should form the major part of the diet; (3) proteins, starches and fats should be eaten in small quantities; (4) only wholegrain and unprocessed starches should be used and all refined processed foods should be taboo, in particular white flour and sugar and all foods made with them, and highly processed fats such as margarine; (5) an interval of at least four to four-and-a-half hours should elapse between meals of different character. The book also includes a chart which is a complete list of the types of foods that can be combined and those combinations which should always be avoided.

In practice I find that Hay's original list can be modified to suit today's lifestyle. He was not an advocate of vegetarian protein, but there are more than 2 million non-meat eaters in Britain and I have found no problems with lentils, beans and other vegetarian foods. Hay also suggests alcohol which is suitable to drink with different meals. This is not something which I recommend except in moderation; we now know more about the long-term dangers of alcohol. For more advice on the Hay diet read *Superfoods and The Superfoods Diet*.

More about additives

We have already seen what can be in a slice of ordinary everyday swiss roll (page 44). Most pre-packed food contains food additives. Yet these additives provide no nutritional value and are only there for the convenience of food manufacturers and retailers. Practitioners of alternative medicine have been warning about the dangers of additives since 1970. It is certain that many asthmatic and allergic children suffer as a result of eating foods containing additives. It's also certain that many non-allergic people suffer some adverse reactions to the chemicals in the food they eat. In spite of what the supporters of food additives say, the majority of these chemicals are not tested nor are they under the control of government departments, and the best advice is to try to avoid them. This is even more important if anyone in your family is known to suffer from allergies. It is only when we, the public, stop buying junk foods that manufacturers will be forced to provide a healthier alternative.

What the E numbers mean

The following is a list of the commonest E numbers and the names of the substances they represent:

E102	Tartrazine	E231 and	
E104	Quinoline yellow	232	Diphenyl derivatives
E107	Yellow 2G	E239	Hexamine
E110	Sunset yellow	E249	Potassium nitrite
E120	Cochineal	E250	Sodium nitrite
E122	Carmoisine	E251	Sodium nitrate
E123	Amaranth	E252	Potassium nitrate (saltpetre)
E124	Ponceau 4R	E261	Potassium acetate
E127	Erythrosine	E262	Sodium acetate
E128	Red 2G	E270	Lactic acid
E131	Patent blue V	E280 to	
E132	Indigo carmine	283	Derivatives of propionic acid
E133	Brilliant blue	E290	Carbon dioxide
E142	Green S	E310	Propyl gallate
E150	Caramel	E311	Octyl gallate
E151	Black PN	E312	Dodecyl gallate
E153	Carbon black	E320	Butylated hydroxyanisole (BHA)
E154	Brown FK		
E155	Brown HT	E321	Butylated hydroxytolene (BHT)
E173	Aluminium		
E174	Silver	E325	Sodium lactate
E175	Gold	E385	Calcium disodium (RDTA)
E180	Pigment rubine	E407	Carrageenan (Irish moss)
E200	Sorbic acid	E414	Gum arabic
E210 to	Benzoic acid and its	E421	Mannitol
219	benzoates	E430	Polyoxyethylene (8 stearate)
E220	Sulphur dioxide	E431	Polyoxyethylene stearate
E221	Sodium sulphite	E434	Polysorbate 40
E222	Sodium bisulphite	E435	Polysorbate 60
E223	Sodium metabisulphite	E436	Polysorbate 65
E224	Potassium metabisulphite	E450B and	
E226	Calcium sulphite	E450C	Diphosphates
E227	Calcium bisulphite	492	Sorbitan tristearate
E230	Biphenyl (or diphenyl)	508	Potassium chloride

510	Ammonium chloride	623	Calcium glutamate
514	Sodium sulphate	627	Sodium guanylate
541	Sodium aluminium		(guanosine)
	phosphate	631	Inosine 5
544	Calcium polyphosphate	635	Sodium 5
545	Ammonium polyphosphate	924	Potassium bromate
621	Monosodium glutamate	925	Chlorine
622	Monopotassium glutamate	925	Chlorine dioxide

Most of us can eat just about any food without any ill effects. However, if we suffer from certain conditions the substances which certain manufacturers add to food to improve its appearance or shelf life can make those conditions worse. In some people food additives can actually cause a variety of illnesses and some additives should certainly be avoided by babies and young children. We should all be aware of the possible dangers and get to know the E numbers and, most importantly, read the labels on food before we buy it. The following chart gives you a list of all those conditions which may be aggravated or even caused by additives. Parents should take special care about the food given to young children and babies. Additives underlined should be avoided. Foods containing the others should not be eaten in large quantities.

Medical conditions caused by or aggravated by food additives

YOUNG CHILDREN: E211 E212 E213 E214 E215 E216 E217 E250 E251 E252 E262 E310 E311 E312 E320 E321 E325 621 627 631 635

BABIES: E249 E250 E251 E252 E262 E270 E310 E311 E312 E320 E321 E325 514 541 621 622 623 627 631 635

If you suffer from one of the conditions below, you should avoid foods containing additives underlined on this list. Be careful not to eat a lot of foods containing the others.

ALLERGIES: E131 E132 E133 E142 E151 E154 E155 E180 E211 E212 E213 E214 E215 E216 E217 E218 E219 E223 E224 E414 E421

ASTHMA: E102 E104 E107 E110 E120 E122 E124 E128 E133 E142 E151 E154 E155 E180 E210 E211 E212 E213 E214 E215 E216 E217 E221 E222 E223 E224 E226 E227 E249 E250 E251 E252 E310 E311 E312 E320 E321

Food intolerance or food allergy? A vexed question

HYPERACTIVITY: **E102 E104 E107 E110 E120 E122 E123 E124 E128 E133 E142 E151 E154 E155 E180 E210 E220 E321**

ECZEMA: **E115 E430 E431**

HAY FEVER: **E102 E104 E107 E110 E120 E122**

HIGH BLOOD PRESSURE: **E132**

MIGRAINE: **E250 E251 E252 E280 E281 E282 E283 621**

KIDNEY TROUBLE: **E173 E174 E175 E261 E430 510 514 541 622**

LIVER TROUBLE: **E310 E311 E312 510**

ASPIRIN SENSITIVITY: **E102 E104 E107 E110 E120 E122 E123 E124 E155 E180 E310 E311 E312**

Some food additives can cause illness in a small number of people. The conditions listed below could be caused by the food you eat, and numbers underlined are more likely to cause problems than the others. If you are concerned about any of these conditions you should, of course, consult your GP.

VOMITING: **E110 E230 E231 E232 E250 E251 E252 E385 E421 E450B E450C 508 544 545 622 924**

VISUAL DISTURBANCE: **E102 E104 E107 E110 E120 E122**

GASTRIC IRRITATION: **E210 E220 E223 E226 E227 E239 E310 E311 E312 508 622**

VITAMIN DEFICIENCY: **E150 E223 E226 E227 E321 924 925**

GENETIC MUTATION: **E154 E239**

URTICARIA (HIVES): **E102 E104 E107 E110 E120 E122 E123 E131 E132 E200 E210 E211 E223 E430 E431**

URINARY PROBLEMS: **E239**

HEADACHES: **621**

MIGRAINE: **621**

REPRODUCTIVE PROBLEMS: **E310 E311 E312**

BREATHING PROBLEMS: **E102 E107 E110 E120 E122 E131 E132**

OEDEMA (SWELLING):	**E110 E122**
SENSITIVITY TO LIGHT:	**E127**
OVERACTIVE THYROID:	**E127**
NAUSEA:	**E131 E132 E230 E231 E232 E250 E251 E252 E421 508 621 622 924**
LOW BLOOD PRESSURE:	**E131 E250 E251 E252**
CANCER (POSSIBLE RISK):	**E153 E239 E249 E250 E251 E252 E407 E434 E435 E436**
SKIN IRRITATION:	**E218 E219 E239**
INCREASED EFFECT OF ALCOHOL:	**E290**
INCREASED CHOLESTEROL LEVEL:	**E321**
ULCERATIVE COLITIS (POSSIBLE RISK):	**E407**
INCREASED ABSORPTION OF FAT-SOLUBLE SUBSTANCES:	**E434 E435 E436 492**
PALPITATIONS:	**621**
DIZZINESS:	**621**
GOUT:	**627 631 635**

A shopper's guide to food additives

Know where to look for the E numbers on the supermarket shelf. You would expect to find some colourings, flavourings and preservatives in most packet and tinned foods on your supermarket shelf, but as the list below shows, many seemingly fresh foods also have those little E numbers lurking in them. Dairy produce like yoghurt, for instance, often contains food colourings which can be particularly bad for some children. Some fish fingers contain artificial colouring, and even citrus fruits and their by-products have often been sprayed with a fungicide and the only way to get this off is by washing the fruit in warm water. So beware the slice of lemon in your gin and tonic, or even in your Perrier water, it could contain up

277

to seventy times the amount of anti-fungal chemical normally allowed in foods.

Shopping guide to food additives

CONFECTIONERY:	**E102 E110 E132 E150 E153 E200 E210–219 E270 E310 E311 E312 E320 E321 E325 E421**
FRESH CITRUS FRUIT:	**E230 E231 E232**
SOFT DRINKS BEER AND CIDER:	**E102 E150 E153 E200 E210–219 E220 E223 E226 E227 E270 E290 E320 E321 E385 E407**
TINNED FOOD:	**E102 E123 E124 E127 E133 E142 E200 E210–219 E220 E250 E251 E252**
CONVENIENCE FOODS:	**E102 E110 E122 E132 E142 E200 E220 E223 E310 E311 E312 E320 E321 621**
DESSERTS:	**E110 E123 E124 E153 E210–219 E220 E407**
PACKET SOUPS:	**E110 E122 E123 E124 E150 E220 621**
MEAT PRODUCTS:	**E104 E127 E128 E131 E150 E220 E249 E250 E251 E252 E450 621**
BAKERY PRODUCTS:	**E110 E122 E123 E124 E127 E132 E142 E150 E151 E173 E174 E175 E200 E210–219 E262 E280–283 E320 E321 E407 E415 E435 492 541 635 924 925**
DAIRY PRODUCTS:	**E102 E110 E180 E200 E210–219 E221 E239 E251 E280–283 E320 E321 E325 E407 E421 E450 544 545**
FISH:	**E102 E104 E154 E220 E259 E450**

Fortunately, pressure from you the consumers of food is forcing more and more retailers, especially the large supermarkets, to offer a wider selection of foods which are free from artificial additives, preservatives, colourings and flavourings. However, be careful as many of the newer packages are very misleading. A large flash on the front of a packet of yoghurt which says 'Free from artificial colours and flavours' can be tempting, but turn the pack over and look at the small print on the bottom. You may well find that it does contain additives and preservatives, while the loaf of bread so appetisingly labelled in bold print 'Free from all artificial colours' may still contain antioxidants. So, learn to be a label reader, and above all encourage your children to do the same. They can't learn good eating habits early enough.

The great debate

Since the early part of this century, the naturopaths have been convinced that food additives, colourings, flavourings, preservatives, sugar, refined carbohydrates, and an increasing proportion of animal protein and animal fats in our diets, have all contributed to the diseases of civilisation which threaten the health of nations. Little by little the open-minded and far-seeing members of the scientific and medical establishments have begun to accept some of these ideas and to look for scientific explanations for them. Within the academic world there is argument and there are those who say that there has been no conclusive and irrefutable proof that food additives cause problems in children, or that animal fats cause heart disease, or that sugar is harmful to the health, or that diets low in natural fibres and high in refined starches are a definite cause of severe digestive disorders. However, there is ample evidence to show that changing the diet to one in which there is more fibre, less fat, less sugar, less salt and less animal protein is beneficial to the health in general and to all the specific areas already mentioned.

The barons of big business are on the defensive since they see their markets threatened. They are spending huge amounts of money on advertising, promotion and propaganda campaigns in order to convince the public that the food freaks like me are a greater threat to people's health than the products of their industries. Depriving children of their sweets is bad for them. Cutting down on fats can reduce their calorie intake. Vegetarianism can lead to vitamin deficiencies. And parents who foist their radical ideas of diet on to their children are at risk of creating muesli belt malnutrition in tens of thousands of children throughout the country. All this is, of course, total nonsense.

Ridiculously extreme or obsessional diets are not healthy, but the vast majority of thinking parents do not need persuading that the youngsters of today are growing up as a junk food generation. Instant meals, takeaways, the inevitable burger and chips, sweetened fizzy drinks, artificially coloured, high fat, high sugar milk shakes, salty, fatty and filling snacks, all these are the real danger to the health of our children. Compared to the rest of Europe, British children eat more sugar, more fat, less fibre, and less fresh fruit and vegetables than those in every other country. This does not bode well for their future health and it will create ever-growing problems for the resources of the British National Health Service.

Every parent has a responsibility to try to encourage healthier patterns of eating in their children. And don't forget that children learn by example. If you live on junk foods it's no good trying to persuade your children to eat their greens. If you're too lazy ever to peel an orange, it's not likely that your children are going to become enthusiastic fruit eaters. It is not necessary to deprive them of treats. There are plenty of alternatives to the tooth-rotting products of the sugar industry, and it's also worth noting that many of the foods with a high sugar content are those with the lowest nutritional value. Too many of these sweet sticky snacks will also fill your children up and displace from their daily diets the more nourishing foods which they need so desperately.

Try to make your children aware of the blandishments of the advertisers, discuss advertisements with them, get them to save food packets, and together look at the labels. Teach them to be suspicious of the claims of individual manufacturers and especially of large trade organisations. A recent video film produced by the sugar industry and distributed to schools as educational material suggests that an apple a day won't keep the dentist away, and may in fact do more harm to teeth than a bar of chocolate. This film, produced by the Sugar Bureau, which represents the industry in Britain, suggests that giving up sugar is an unrealistic measure and further that sugar is not the main cause of tooth decay.

The Health Education Council took the unprecedented step of writing to every Educational Authority advising them not to show this film in their schools and the British Dental Association described the film as 'a grossly misleading and deliberate attempt to minimise the dangers done to teeth by sugars'.

Don't be swayed by the purveyors of ill-health. Use your own judgement and your own common sense to choose a sensible and balanced diet for you and your family. You do not have to become a food freak, you do not have to become a vegetarian, a vegan or a macrobiotic eater. All you need is moderation. As a simple rule of thumb, try to make one-third of your daily food intake fresh, raw produce – fruits, salads and vegetables. Get more of your protein from fish and poultry. Cut down on the animal fats by avoiding meat products such as pies, pasties, sausages, salamis, ham, bacon and pâtés. Cut down on sugar, cut down on salt. Increase the amount of wholegrain cereals you eat, wholemeal bread, brown rice, wholemeal pasta – these are all healthy, cheap and nutritious. Try to make more use of vegetarian sources of protein such as beans, lentils and nuts. Use dried fruits and fruit juices as natural forms of sweetening. Avoid the frying pan. When you do cook vegetables, either steam them or cook them for as short a time as possible in as little water as possible and then add the water to gravies or soups, so that you do not lose the valuable minerals or vitamins.

If you're not satisfied with the food served to your children at school, or to yourselves at work, complain and if all else fails, take your own lunches, or make your children healthy packed lunches, and encourage others to do the same. There is nothing like a drop in turnover and consequent loss of profit to make caterers improve the quality of the food they serve.

We are what we eat, and there is no doubt that the seeds of coronary heart disease are sown during childhood. So, don't encourage your children to dig their graves with their teeth.

Booklist

The Women's Guide to Homeopathy, Dr Andrew Lockie, published by Hamish Hamilton.

Food Combining for Health, Doris Grant and Jean Joyce, published by Thorsons.

E for Additives, Maurice Hanssen, published by Thorsons.

Traveller's Health, Richard Dawood, published by OUP.

Superfoods and The Superfoods Diet, Michael van Straten and Barbara Griggs, published by Dorling Kindersley.

Zest for Life, Barbara Griggs, published by Ebury Press.

The Family Guide to Food and Health, Elizabeth Morse, John Rivers and Anne Heughen, published by Barrie and Jenkins.

The Complete Manual of Organic Gardening, Basil Caplan, published by Headline.

Homeopathy for Mother and Baby, Miranda Castro, published by Macmillan.

Useful addresses

For information about acupuncture, chiropractic, homoeopathy, medical herbalism, naturopathy and osteopathy contact:

The Council for Complementary and Alternative Medicine (CCAM)
179 Gloucester Place
London NW1 6DX
Tel: 071–724 9103

The General Council and Register of Naturopaths
6 Netherhall Gardens
London NW3 5RR
Tel: 071–435 6464

The British Acupuncture Association
34 Alderney Street
London SW1V 4EV
Tel: 071–834 1012

The Society of Teachers of the Alexander Technique
Suite 20
10 London House
266 Fulham Road
London SW10 9EL
Tel: 071–351 0828

The British Chiropractic Association
Premiere House
10 Greycoat Place
London SW1P 1SB
Tel: 071–222 8866

National Institute of Medical Herbalists
9 Palace Gate
Exeter
Devon EX1 1JA
Tel: 0392 426022

The General Council and Register of Osteopaths
56 London Road
Reading
Berkshire RG1 4SQ
Tel: 0734 576585

The Disabled Living Foundation
380 Harrow Road
London W9 2HG
Tel: 081–289 6111

The Cancer Help Centre
Grove House
Cornwallis Grove
Clifton
Bristol BS8 4PG
Tel: 0272 743216

The Vegetarian Society
Parkdale
Dunham Road
Altrincham
Cheshire WA14 4QG
Tel: 061–928 0793

Useful addresses

Homoeopathic remedies from:

Ainsworths
38 New Cavendish Street
London W1M 7LH
Tel: 071–935 5330

Index

Index

Sexual Awareness

Enhancing Sexual Pleasure

Barry and Emily McCarthy

ILLUSTRATED   NEW UNEXPURGATED EDITION

This book is written to show individuals and couples how to enhance their sexual pleasure. It is focused on feelings and fulfilment, and emphasizes a joyful expression of sexuality and intimacy.

The path to a new awareness includes chapters on:
The Pleasure of Touching
Self-Exploration
Increasing Arousal For Women
Becoming Orgasmic
Learning Control
Overcoming Inhibition

With the current emphasis on the importance of just one sexual partner, this is a timely publication designed to show you just how to make the most of that relationship, and how to build a new sexual partnership.

NON-FICTION/REFERENCE   0 7472 3561 9

More Health and Fitness Non-Fiction from Headline:

Miriam Stoppard

LOSE 7lbs IN 7 DAYS
AND BE SLIM AND HEALTHY
FOR THE REST OF YOUR LIFE

Do you want to lose a little weight for a special
occasion? Are your clothes getting a bit too tight? Or
do you simply want to be fitter, healthier and slimmer?

With this delicious, easy and simple eating plan, I
show you how to lose weight without spending lots of
money on expensive food. What's more, I make sure
that you need never go hungry as I *insist* that you eat
SIX times a day.

Better still, since I believe that dieting should be fun,
not a mild form of purgatory, I show you how to
pamper yourself and enjoy life whilst continuing to
lose weight.

Finally, I provide lots of advice, based on my own
experience both as a doctor and as a lifelong dieter,
on how to keep up the good work once you've shed
those pounds.

Too good to be true? Try it and see. It works!

Based on the bestselling video
released through Virgin

NON-FICTION/HEALTH   0 7472 3565 1

More bestselling non fiction from Headline

THE MURDER YEARBOOK	Brian Lane	£5.99□
THE ENCYCLOPAEDIA OF SERIAL KILLERS	Brian Lane & Wilfred Gregg	£6.99 □
ONE LIFETIME IS NOT ENOUGH	Zsa Zsa Gabor	£5.99 □
GINGER: My Story	Ginger Rogers	£6.99 □
MICROWAVE GOURMET	Barbara Kafka	£5.99 □
PLAYFAIR CRICKET ANNUAL 1992	Bill Frindall	£2.99 □
PLAYFAIR FOOTBALL ANNUAL 1992-93	Jack Rollin	£3.99 □
DEBRETT'S CORRECT FORM	Patrick Montague-Smith	£7.99 □
DEBRETT'S ETIQUETTE & MODERN MANNERS	Elsie Burch Donald	£7.99 □
SUNDAY EXPRESS GENERAL KNOWLEDGE CROSSWORD BOOK Volume 1	*Sunday Express*	£2.99 □

All Headline books are available at your local bookshop or newsagent, or can be ordered direct from the publisher. Just tick the titles you want and fill in the form below. Prices and availability subject to change without notice.

Headline Book Publishing PLC, Cash Sales Department, Bookpoint, 39 Milton Park, Abingdon, OXON, OX14 4TD, UK. If you have a credit card you may order by telephone — 0235 831700.

Please enclose a cheque or postal order made payable to Bookpoint Ltd to the value of the cover price and allow the following for postage and packing:
UK & BFPO: £1.00 for the first book, 50p for the second book and 30p for each additional book ordered up to a maximum charge of £3.00.
OVERSEAS & EIRE: £2.00 for the first book, £1.00 for the second book and 50p for each additional book.

Name ....

Address ....

....

....

If you would prefer to pay by credit card, please complete:
Please debit my Visa/Access/Diner's Card/American Express (delete as applicable) card no:

Signature ....Expiry Date ....